# Supporting Survivors of Sexual Violence and Abuse

T0299782

This textbook provides practical guidance to enable health professionals to support survivors of sexual violence. It gives insight into the complex and wide-ranging nature and experience of sexual violence, barriers to disclosure, and explores the implications for survivors, health professionals and healthcare organisations.

An evidence-based resource, this book provides information, guidance and signposting for all those who might receive disclosures of sexual violence, challenging perceptions, stigma and judgement. As well as discussing disclosure of recent experiences, it takes into account that life events may trigger the re-surfacing of prior experiences. The book also operates as a practical tool, prompting professionals to reflect on their own clinical experience of dealing with disclosures of sexual violence. The chapters look at the full breadth of sexual violence and abuse, including rape and sexual assault, child sexual abuse, harassment and stalking, exploitation, trafficking, conflict situations, traditional practices and sexual violence in LGBTQAI+ communities.

Enabling readers to develop the necessary knowledge and understanding to inform their practice, this book is a comprehensive resource for all health professionals, across primary and secondary care. It is also a valuable text for those taking post-registration courses in sexual health, specialist community and public health nursing, district nursing, mental health and children's nursing among others. Reflection sections can be used to support professional registration revalidation.

**Claire Dosdale** is an Assistant Professor in the Department of Nursing, Midwifery and Health at Northumbria University, UK. She has worked as both a clinical specialist nurse and a lecturer practitioner, in sexual health. She currently teaches pre-registration nursing and safeguarding, sexual health, sexual violence to post-qualifying healthcare students. Her research focuses on supporting survivors of sexual violence in healthcare and workplace experiences of sexual harassment and sexual assault.

**Emma Senior** is an Assistant Professor in the Department of Nursing, Midwifery and Health at Northumbria University, UK. She teaches, among other things, sexual health, safeguarding and public health to post-registration students.

**Lynette Shotton** is an Associate Professor in the Department of Social Work, Education and Community Well-being, Northumbria University, UK, with a professional background in adult nursing and health visiting. Her current role is primarily concerned with academic leadership and her research interests are focused on understanding and addressing health and educational inequality.

**Katy Skarparis** is an Assistant Professor in the Department of Nursing, Midwifery and Health at Northumbria University, UK. She has a background in behaviour change research and has a special interest in the area of sexual violence. She currently teaches safeguarding in the area of sexual violence to pre- and post-registration healthcare students.

# Supporting Survivors of Sexual Violence and Abuse

## Approaches to Care for Health Professionals

**Claire Dosdale, Emma Senior, Lynette Shotton and Katy Skarparis**

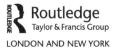
Routledge
Taylor & Francis Group

LONDON AND NEW YORK

Designed cover image: Routledge

First published 2024
by Routledge
4 Park Square, Milton Park, Abingdon, Oxon OX14 4RN

and by Routledge
605 Third Avenue, New York, NY 10158

*Routledge is an imprint of the Taylor & Francis Group, an informa business*

*British Library Cataloguing-in-Publication Data*
Names: Dosdale, Claire, author. | Senior, Emma, author. | Shotton, Lynette, author. | Skarparis, Katy, author.
Title: Supporting survivors of sexual violence and abuse : approaches to care for health professionals / Claire Dosdale, Emma Senior, Lynette Shotton and Katy Skarparis.
Description: Abingdon, Oxon ; New York, NY : Routledge, 2024. | Includes bibliographical references and index
Identifiers: LCCN 2023045190 | ISBN 9781032126241 (hardback) | ISBN 9781032126227 (paperback) | ISBN 9781003225461 (ebook)
Subjects: LCSH: Sexual abuse victims--Services for.
Classification: LCC HV6625 .D673 2024 | DDC 362.883/8--dc23/eng/20240117
LC record available at https://lccn.loc.gov/2023045190

ISBN: 978-1-032-12624-1 (hbk)
ISBN: 978-1-032-12622-7 (pbk)
ISBN: 978-1-003-22546-1 (ebk)

DOI: 10.4324/9781003225461

Typeset in Sabon LT Pro
by KnowledgeWorks Global Ltd.

Access the Support Material: www.routledge.com/9781032126241

# Contents

*List of Tables*                                                                                     *vi*
*Acknowledgements*                                                                                   *vii*

1  Introduction to Book                                                                                1

2  Sexual Violence and Abuse                                                                           7

3  Disclosures of Sexual Violence and Abuse                                                           19

4  Sexual Assault, Sexual Harassment and Stalking                                                     32

5  Trafficking of People for the Purpose of Sexual Exploitation                                       49

6  Child Sexual Abuse                                                                                 62

7  Sexual Violence and Abuse in Marginalised Communities                                             79

8  Supporting Survivors of Sexual Violence and Abuse                                                  95

9  Practitioner Guidance in Supporting Survivors of Sexual Violence
   and Abuse                                                                                         110

10 Reflective Journal                                                                                124

   *Index*                                                                                           *128*

# Tables

| | | |
|---|---|---|
| 3.1 | Example of Rape Myths | 21 |
| 4.1 | Stalking: Types of Survivors | 35 |
| 4.2 | Stalking: Types of Perpetrators | 36 |
| 8.1 | Principles of Trauma-Informed Approaches | 100 |
| 8.2 | Medical Considerations Following Sexual Violence and Abuse | 104 |
| 8.3 | Legal Responsibilities in Reporting Disclosures of Sexual Violence and Abuse | 106 |
| 9.1 | NHS Staff Survey Data in Relation to Burnout | 112 |

# Acknowledgements

Most healthcare practitioners are not adequately prepared to support survivors of sexual violence and abuse. It is not a topic that is prioritised or receives much focus in pre-qualifying education and training; however, it is one of the biggest contributors to health, health inequalities and the well-being of our nation. We hope this book provides a direction for those who might need it. This book could not have been written without all the years of work survivors, academics, activists and practitioners have been doing to improve the lives of those experiencing abuse, and the work towards eradicating sexual violence. Thank you.

# 1 Introduction to Book

## Introduction

Sexual violence and abuse (SVA) is the general term used to describe the process and commission of manipulating or forcing another individual into an unwanted sexual act(s) or activity(ies) without their consent (Rape Crisis, 2022). SVA is committed disproportionately against women and girls, with the perpetrators being overwhelmingly men, and as such, you may find this book focuses mainly on SVA and abuse against women and girls. We have, however, tried to incorporate everyone's experiences of SVA.

Any behaviour of a sexual nature that takes place without consent and produces distress for the person experiencing it is considered to be SVA. It must be noted that consent may be impeded by ability to exercise choice, age, illness, disability, mental capacity, fear and/or alcohol or other drug use. SVA includes (but is not limited to) rape (as well as attempted rape) and also includes unwanted sexual touching, sexual harassment, child sexual abuse and exploitation, female genital mutilation (FGM), taking or sharing sexual images or videos without consent, forced marriage, trafficking of people for the purpose of exploitation and conflict-related SVA. SVA is often situated within a wider context of gender-based violence against women. It is worth noting that all countries have their own legal definition of SVA that is specific for certain types of SVA, and some types are not recognised in a range of countries as SVA within the realms of the law. This book is written and published from a UK perspective; however, understanding the laws relating to your region of practice is essential in supporting survivors.

SVA is a significant violation of human rights; a deeply violating and painful experience for the survivor with both immediate and long-term health implications, which include physical, sexual, mental and reproductive health problems, as well as social and economic costs resulting from inability to work and lack of participation in activities of daily living, including caring for themselves and their children and families (World Health Organisation [WHO], 2021). In the UK alone, it is estimated that rape and other sexual offences cost the economy approximately £12.2bn per year (Heeks et al., 2018). As such, SVA is an increasingly serious public health concern. Whilst SVA is not discriminatory of age, sex, religion, race, social status or class, SVA is a gender-based violence, with women being significantly more at risk than men (Borumandnia et al., 2020). Several research papers have studied SVA prevalence in specific sub-communities, which adds to the difficulty of defining the overall global picture of the prevalence of all types of SVA; however, Borumandnia et al. (2020) recently explored the overall prevalence of SVA and found that SVA statistics continue to show higher prevalence in women, as opposed to men in both high- and low-income countries.

DOI: 10.4324/9781003225461-1

Statistics on SVA are difficult to ascertain. This is due to a range of factors which include underreporting, lack of adequate recording of incidences when they are disclosed, attrition rates of cases, disbelieving attitudes and exclusion of large pockets of the population in most studies, specifically older people and those identified with specific vulnerabilities. Consequently, it is impossible to accurately measure the prevalence of SVA amongst the population. As a result, statistics surrounding SVA are acknowledged to be vastly underestimated and as such should be interpreted with caution. Increased recording of these statistics is becoming more common and whilst this has begun to give a greater insight of the scale of *all* types of SVA in the world today, it is clear, that far more people experience incidences of SVA than will ever report (Ceelen et al., 2019; Office of National Statistics [ONS], 2023).

In the UK, it is suggested 4.880 million women and 989,000 men have experienced some form of SVA since the age of 16 (ONS, 2021); this equates to 1:4 women and 1:20 men. Worldwide it is estimated that 1:3 women have experienced SVA; male statistics are more difficult to ascertain. Survivorsuk.org (2021) suggests that an estimated 12,000 men are raped in the UK every year, and more than 70,000 are sexually abused or assaulted yearly. SVA experience in men is underreported making it difficult to estimate prevalence. SVA against men is less understood and/or acknowledged in some cultures. Gender norms combined with cultural and religious taboos contribute to underreporting of male SVA.

When considering specific offences, it is evident that reported rape offences in the UK have increased dramatically in the past 18 years; with 18,400 incidences reported in 2012/2013 compared to 62,200 in 2019/2020 (ONS, 2020) and 70,633 in 2023 (ONS, 2023). It is important to note that only 5–15% of survivors report SVA; 5:6 women who are raped and 4:5 men who experience rape do not report (Brooker and Durmaz, 2015; ONS, 2021); these statics run the risk of becoming phenomenal when considering those who do not report/tell. Thus, demonstrating the need of support for these survivors.

The COVID-19 pandemic saw a perfect storm for SVA. Many people were at home with their abusers and access to services in order to disclose or seek guidance was limited. As communities around the world faced unprecedented uncertainty to follow their governments' guidance to stay at home and/or reduce contact with friends and family, women and girls were placed at heightened risk of domestic violence, intimate partner violence, child abuse, and other forms of sexual and gender-based violence. It should be noted that lockdown may have also provided a protective effect for some of those experiencing or who are at risk of SVA from someone they do not live with (e.g., a non-cohabiting partner, or travel restrictions in the case of FGM, sexual trafficking or forced marriage). As lockdown and restrictions are removed (they are removed at the time of publishing), it is likely these risks will again rise (Dosdale and Skarparis, 2021).

Sexual harassment, rape culture and assault claims made by school pupils on the website 'Everyone's Invited' (2021) have been the current focus of many child abuse scandals to engulf the nation and contribute to many ongoing globally. The National Crime Agency (2021) suggests that 1:6 children are sexually abused, and since 2013, they have seen referral of child abuse images up by 1000%. The UK government anticipated a surge in child abuse reporting as the nation came out of lockdown; this should be of global concern. With this, vast majorities of schools, colleges and universities took measures to improve their safeguarding responsibilities by putting an increasing focus on tacking SVA.

As the number of reported incidents of SVA increases, so does the likelihood of practitioners' experiencing disclosure within the healthcare setting, but also, and importantly, caring for an individual who may have experienced SVA, but is yet to disclose. This is where our relationship-building skills are essential to create opportunities for survivors to disclose and receive support. Healthcare practitioners' (HCPs) roles are continually evolving, leading to an increase in responsibility (particularly with advanced clinical management) meaning, HCPs are significantly more likely to receive and manage disclosures of SVA. It is here where this book has relevance, seeking to equip HCPs with the knowledge and skills to provide evidence-based practice in supporting survivors of SVA and to compliment wider professional training and practice.

HCPs are educated and trained to have the ability to recognise signs and symptoms of illness, disease, deterioration and to respond with increased focus on improving health outcomes. For example, 1:16 people in the UK have diabetes (Diabetes UK, 2023); there are clear national frameworks for the management of this condition. What is concerning is that the statistics of 1:3 women who are known to have experienced SVA far outweigh prevalence for other health issues, yet there is little national guidance on identification, management and specialist education for practitioners to aid in supporting survivors. Those most likely to receive disclosures of SVA are thought to be those who work in sexual health services, emergency departments, and GP community care and walk-in centres. However, a disclosure or indicators of SVA could be identified within any area of health and social care where a therapeutic relationship has been built, whether in an acute or community setting. When considering the number of potential survivors, the implications of this disclosure on health and well-being, from both the survivor's perspective and health services, are considerable.

SVA-associated post-traumatic stress (PTS) is a significant public health concern due to the substantial ongoing health implications for the survivor. These include anxiety, stress, fear, nervousness, social isolation, flashbacks, sleeping difficulties, drug/alcohol reliance, low self-esteem, self-harm and suicide. Enhancing what happens before, during and after disclosure within a healthcare setting may provide greater support for the survivors and have a positive impact on recovery. Whilst the forensic evidence is incredibly important to convict an assailant, if the initial disclosure of SVA is not managed with sensitivity, skill and knowledge, the case will rarely get as far as the survivor reaching a Sexual Assault Referral Centre (SARC) in order for forensic samples and assessment to be performed. Unfortunately, forensic evidence is an essential component to improve the likelihood of conviction, and conviction is unfortunately a major component of aiding recovery (Dunmore, Clark and Ehlers, 1999). Whilst this route must always be a choice, research indicates that survivors have better psychological outcomes when they see their assailant brought to justice (Starzynski et al., 2005; Home Office, 2010).

UK policy drivers (Department of Health [DoH], 2001; Home Office, 2010; Department of Health [DoH], 2012; Department of Health [DoH], 2013; ONS, 2013; Crown Prosecution Service (CPS), 2019; Health Scotland, 2019) consistently seem to specify that HCPs must encourage disclosures of SVA to both improve the emotional support for survivors at the earliest possible stage and to aid in increasing conviction rates for perpetrators of SVA. Evidence suggests survivor's negative experiences of these initial disclosures in the healthcare setting continue to have a detrimental impact on health and well-being (Ahrens et al., 2007; Campbell, 2008; McTavish et al., 2019). Furthermore, evidence also indicates that once a survivor has made an initial disclosure of SVA, the response of the person disclosed to is fundamental in reducing the psychological sequelae and the incidence of PTS (Ullman, 1999; Starzynski et al., 2005; Starzynski et al., 2007; Ahrens, Cabral and Abeling, 2009; Home Office, 2010). Westmarland, Alderson and Kirkham (2012) acknowledge this and propose therapeutic interventions (if received as early as possible following the experience) can prevent the onset of chronic PTS. It is therefore of the upmost importance that HCPs 'get this right'. This book aims to provide a resource to aid HCPs in supporting survivors of all forms of SVA and in all clinical contexts.

This book aims to provide a resource to aid HCPs in supporting survivors of all forms of SVA and in all clinical contexts. As mentioned at the beginning of this chapter, SVA is committed disproportionately against women and girls, with the perpetrators being overwhelmingly men, and as such, you may find this book focuses mainly on SVA and abuse against women and girls. We have, however, tried to incorporate everyone's experiences of SVA.

## What to Expect throughout This Book

**Chapter 2 – Sexual Violence and Abuse:** this chapter aims to further explore the term 'SVA'. It will explore more in-depth the types of SVA and how these have evolved (or not) over time. The impact of SVA and the burden of health will also be explored.

Chapter 3 – **Disclosures of Sexual Violence and Abuse:** this chapter will explore the notion of victim blaming, rape myths, unconscious bias and the impact this has on survivors of SVA. It will critically explore disclosure – who people disclose to, the response in both the social and formal setting and the impact of the response. This will be followed by a more in-depth exploration regarding the affect SVA disclosure can have on both psychological and physical well-being.

### Chapters 4–7

*The following four chapters are exploring types of SVA in more depth. In each of these chapters you will find further in-depth information regarding the focus topic.*

Chapter 4 – **Sexual Assault, Sexual Harassment and Stalking:** This chapter will also touch upon these three types of SVA. There will be a focus on violence against women and girls in this chapter. As technology evolves so does the means for someone to find themselves being sexually harassed and stalked digitally. This chapter will explore how the digital world is used for this type of SVA and what that means for the individual.

Chapter 5 – **Trafficking of People for the Purpose of Sexual Exploitation:** This chapter will not only define sexual exploitation in relation to trafficking but also explore the varied ways this can be executed.

Chapter 6 – **Child Sexual Abuse:** This chapter will explore the definition of child sexual abuse; it will provide an in-depth review of when and how children may disclose by exploring potential behaviour patterns that may lead to identification of abuse. The chapter will explore ways in which to support children once a disclosure is made.

Chapter 7 – **Sexual Violence and Abuse in Marginalised Communities:** This chapter will introduce SVA in armed conflict and traditional practices (including FGM/forced marriage/so-called honour-based abuse). It will also explore the use of SVA in ritual communities. At times, the need of those experiencing these types of SVA can vastly differ from others. It is important to explore some of these communities in more depth, especially considering the impact on health and well-being and engagement with services.

Chapter 8 – **Supporting Survivors of Sexual Violence and Abuse:** This chapter focuses on the psychological impact of disclosures, specifically how trauma effects the survivors and the direct impact this has on health. Trauma-informed care and practice are explored alongside the practical elements of support such as communication skills, STI and pregnancy risk, signposting and forensic medical examinations/informing others.

Chapter 9 – **Practitioner Guidance in Supporting Survivors of Sexual Violence and Abuse:** In this chapter we explore some of the legal and safeguarding frameworks you may need when supporting survivors of SVA. It will also emphasise essential need for staff to access support after working with survivors of SVA due to the highly emotive nature. The emotional impact on staff is neglected in practice; however, it should not be underestimated, for many reasons. Consequences of supporting survivors include anxiety, concern/worry, fear of legal impact, burnout, and the potential of re-living own experiences of trauma or that of friends and family. This chapter explores the responsibility of the HCP in the court proceedings. It will give guidance on writing a statement for criminal cases and presenting that statement in a court of law, as a professional witness.

Chapter 10 – **Reflective Journal:** This chapter allows space for reflection on your learning. There is a structured reflective journal space for use in practice – this is aligned with the Nursing & Midwifery Council/General Medical Council reflection documentation to use for revalidation purposes and can also be used with the Continuing to Fitness to Practice process for members of the Health Professionals Council.

## References

Ahrens, C. E., Cabral, G. and Abeling, S. (2009) 'Healing or hurtful: Sexual assault survivor's interpretations of social reactions from support providers', *Psychology of Women Quarterly*, 33(1), pp. 81–94.

Ahrens, C. E., Campbell, R., Ternier-Themes, N., Wasco, S. M. and Sefl, T. (2007) 'Deciding whom to tell: Expectations and outcomes of rape survivors' first disclosures', *Psychology of Women's Quarterly*, 31, pp. 38–49.

Borumandnia, N., Khadembashi, N., Tabatabaei, M. and Majd, A. H. (2020) 'The prevalence rate of sexual violence worldwide: A trend analysis', *BMC Public Health* 20, p. 1835. https://doi.org/10.1186/s12889-020-09926-5

Brooker, C. and Durmaz, E. (2015) 'Mental health, sexual violence and the work of sexual assault referral centres (SARCs) in England', *Journal of Forensic and Legal Medicine*, 37, pp. 47–51. https://doi.org/10.1016/j.jflm.2015.01.006

Campbell, R. (2008) 'The psychological impact of rape', *American Psychologist*, 63(8), pp. 702–717.

Ceelen, M., Dorn, T., Flora, S., van Huis, F. S. and Reijnders, U. J. L. (2019) 'Characteristics and post-decision attitudes of non-reporting sexual violence victims', *Journal of Interpersonal Violence*, 34(9), pp. 1961–1977.

Crown Prosecution Service (CPS) (2019) *Violence Against Women and Girls Report 2019*. Available at: https://www.cps.gov.uk/sites/default/files/documents/publications/cps-vawg-report-2019.pdf

Department of Health (DoH) (2001) *Better Prevention, Better Services, Better Sexual Health – A National Strategy for Sexual Health and HIV*. Available at: https://extranet.who.int/country planningcycles/sites/default/files/planning_cycle_repository/united_kingdom/hiv_plan_uk.pdf

Department of Health (DoH) (2012) *Protecting People, Promoting Health: A Public Health Approach to Violence Prevention in England*. Available at: http://www.nwph.net/nwpho/Publications/Protecting%20People%20Promoting%20Health%20Web.pdf

Department of Health (DoH) (2013) *A Framework for Sexual Health Improvement for England*. Available at: https://www.gov.uk/government/publications/a-framework-for-sexual-health-improvement-in-england

Diabetes UK (2023) *Diabetes Prevalence[vedio]*https://www.diabetes.co.uk/diabetes-prevalence.html

Dosdale, C. and Skarparis, K. (2021) 'Supporting survivors of sexual violence and abuse during the COVID-19 pandemic', *British Journal of Nursing*, 29(20), pp. 1159–1163.

Dunmore, E., Clark, D. M. and Ehlers, A. (1999) 'Cognitive factors involved in the onset and maintenance of posttraumatic stress disorder (PTSD) after physical or sexual assault', *Behaviour Research and Therapy*, 37(9), pp. 809–829. https://doi.org/10.1016/S0005-7967(98)00181-8

Health Scotland (2019) *Gender Based Violence, Rape and Sexual Assault – What Health Workers Need To Know*. Available at: http://www.healthscotland.scot/publications/gender-based-violence-rape-and-sexual-assault-what-health-workers-need-to-know

Heeks, M., Reed, S., Tasfiri, M. and Prince, S. (2018). *The Economic and Social Costs of Crime*. London: Home Office.

Home Office. (2010) *A Report by Baroness Stern CBE of an Independent Review into How Rape Complainants Are Handled by the Public Authorities in England and Wales*. Available: https://webarchive.nationalarchives.gov.uk/ukgwa/20100418065537/http:/equalities.gov.uk/PDF/Stern_Review_acc_FINAL.pdf

National Crime Agency, (2021) National and Strategic Assessment of Serious and Organised Crime. Available:https://www.nationalcrimeagency.gov.uk/who-we-are/publications/533-national-strategic-assessment-of-serious-and-organised-crime-2021/file

McTavish, J. R., Sverdlichenko, I., MacMillan, H. L. and Welerle, C. (2019) 'Child sexual abuse, disclosure and PTSD: A systematic and critical review', *Child Abuse and Neglect*, 92, pp. 198–208.

Office of National Statistics (ONS) (2013) *An Overview of Sexual Offending in England and Wales*. Available at: https://assets.publishing.service.gov.uk/media/5a7ca66d40f0b65b3de0a47d/sexual-offending-overview-jan-2013.pdf

Office of National Statistics (ONS) (2020) *Sexual Offences in England and Wales Overview*. Available at: https://www.ons.gov.uk/peoplepopulationandcommunity/crimeandjustice/bulletins/sexualoffencesinenglandandwalesoverview/march2020

Office of National Statistics (ONS) (2021) *Crime Survey for England and Wales*. Available at: https://www.ons.gov.uk/peoplepopulationandcommunity/crimeandjustice/bulletins/crimeinengland andwales/yearendingmarch2022#:~:text=Police%20recorded%20crime%20in%20England,2020%20(6.1%20million%20offences)

Office of National Statistics (2023) *Crime in England and Wales: Year Ending Sept 2022* https://www.ons.gov.uk/peoplepopulationandcommunity/crimeandjustice/bulletins/crimeinengland andwales/yearendingseptember2022

Rape Crisis (2022) *Statistics About Sexual Violence and Abuse*. Available at: https://rapecrisis.org.uk/get-informed/statistics-sexual-violence/

Starzynski, L. L., Ullman, S. E., Filipas, H. H. and Townsend, S. M. (2005) 'Correlates of woman's sexual assault disclosure to informal and formal support services', *Violence and Victims*, 20(4), pp. 417–431.

Starzynski, L. L., Ullman, S. E., Townsend, S. M., Long, L. M. and Long, S. M. (2007) 'What factors predict women's disclosure of sexual assault to mental health professionals', *Journal of Community Psychology*, 35(5), pp. 619–638.

SurvivorsUK.org (2021) *Men Overcoming Sexual Violence Together*. Available at: https://www.survivorsuk.org/about-us/#section-1

Ullman, S. E. (1999) 'Social support and recovery from sexual assault: A review', *Aggression and Violent Behaviour*, 4(3), pp. 343–358.

Westmarland, N., Alderson, S. and Kirkham, L. (2012) *The Health, Mental Health And Well-Being Benefits Of Rape Crisis Counselling*. Durham: Durham University and Northern Rock Foundation.

World Health Organisation (WHO) (2021) *Violence Against Women*. Available at: https://www.who.int/news-room/fact-sheets/detail/violence-against-women

# 2 Sexual Violence and Abuse

## Introduction to Chapter

The purpose of this chapter is to present an overview of sexual violence and abuse (SVA) in a little more depth. SVA is a topic not regularly explored within a day-to-day healthcare context, as such, it is not always well understood and may mean different things to different people based on their own experiences with SVA and their societal influences.

Violence against women and girls (VAWG) is a cause and consequence of gender inequality further compounded by intersecting characteristics such as ethnicity, disability, social class, sexuality, gender identity, economic situation, immigration status and age (End Violence Against Women [EVAW], 2022a). As such SVA and VAWG are experienced as a continuum of violence across the life course, which cannot be disaggregated from these inter-connected characteristics and circumstances.

## Definitions and Terminology

Research and literature in general, confusingly, uses a variety of terms interchangeably to describe types of SVA, often referring to one type by three or four different terms. For example, SVA, sexual violence, sexual assault, rape and sexual victimisation are all used as descriptive terms of a 'non-consensual sexual act'. The Crime Survey for England and Wales (Crime Survey of England and Wales [CSEW], 2021) uses the term sexual assault to describe all types of sexual offences recorded by their survey. However, the police use the term sexual assault to record one type of sexual offence (that being the touching of a person without their consent), which is the legal definition (Sexual Offences Act, 2003). In view of this complexity SVA will be used throughout this book as an overarching term incorporating all types of sexual violence.

According to the Ministry of Justice (2022), SVA includes but is not limited to: rape; child sexual abuse; sexual assault; sexual abuse (this includes being coerced into sexual activity you do not want to do); sexual exploitation; image-based sexual abuse; grooming for sexual purposes; female genital mutilation and sexual harassment and stalking (both online and offline). It is important to emphasise the unwanted nature of this activity and that it takes place without consent and/or with the use of coercion. All forms of SVA are serious and it is vital that the person who is/has experienced any form of SVA is not blamed and is supported to understand that it was not their fault; blame is always with the perpetrator and never with the survivor (The Survivors Trust, 2022).

DOI: 10.4324/9781003225461-2

## People Who Have Experienced SVA – Terms Used

One of the most sensitive discussions regarding terminology within the field of SVA is how practitioners/writers/researchers refer to people who have experienced SVA. The four terms used interchangeably throughout literature are as follows: victim, survivor, victim-survivor and complainant. Complainant is used in some research, mostly that which focuses specifically on reporting the SVA to the police. In this context the term complainant is used as a legal term where the individual is considered a complainant of SVA. Due to the vast numbers who do not report their experience to the police, the term complainant will not be used throughout this book.

The term survivor increasingly seems to be the adjective used, due to the association with strength, recovery, empowerment, and the experience of having moved on from the rape (Holstein and Miller, 1990; Thompson, 2000; Parker and Mahlstedt, 2010). It could be argued, however, that this implies that a person has somewhat recovered from their assault (Horvath and Brown, 2022), which may not be the case and could impact individuals seeking support due to the perceived meaning of the term.

Victim was the term used most frequently, but this has been used less so in the last ten years. Thompson's (2000) research demonstrated an association of perceptions of weakness, powerless and vulnerability for women who have experienced rape when the term rape victim was used. However, in the literal sense, victim as a person harmed by criminal acts is an accurate description; the term emphasising the enormity of the experience. Hockett and Saucier (2015) carried out a systematic literature review to explore the two most commonly used terms (victims and survivor) in order to establish the implications for theory, research and recovery. In general, they found that literature exploring rape victims focused on negative outcomes, whilst the rape survivor literature emphasised positive outcomes. Patterson and Campbell (2010) used the term survivor throughout their research to refer to women who had been raped, except when referring to the rape itself and social victimisation (victim-blaming and rape myth adherence). Then, they used the term victim. Guerette and Caron (2007) use both terms throughout their research stating, 'in choosing how to classify herself, a woman has the power to choose how to label a very disempowering experience' (p. 47). Conversely, an SVA survivor is both a victim of a crime and a survivor of that crime. Therefore, the term victim-survivor is often used in current discourse.

The discussion above clearly indicates that there are times when one term is appropriate, times when the other is more acceptable, and times when neither term is appropriate. Many of those who have experienced SVA see themself as both survivor and victim, and neither, at different periods of their post-SVA experience. For consistency, in this book we will use Survivor. However, when supporting people who have experienced SVA, just as you do with all service users, you will be using their name they prefer you to address them as. For any documentation whereby terminology is needed, it is important to ask the survivor which they would like you to use.

## Historical Context

It is suggested that for as long as people have been recording human activity and history, examples of SVA appear. For example, Greek Historians indicate that Alexander the Great was raped by his father-in-law's servants; the use of SVA is illustrated in ancient texts, including Homer's Iliad and the Old Testament of the Holy Bible (Lois, 2021). However, the incidence, motivation and response to SVA vary considerably, as does the meaning of and social tolerance of SVA, which is heavily influenced by the cultural assumptions of time and place.

Studying the history of SVA presents several challenges. Notably, the variation in how SVA is viewed, identified and addressed between and within countries means that the documented evidence is limited. However, recent historical scholarship on the subject focuses primarily on three different sources: established laws, actual cases documented in judicial records and other sources of public record, which include how SVA is represented in popular culture. What is evident that much of the literature focuses on women as victims and men as perpetrators.

In Western nations it is asserted that SVA laws can be traced back to Jewish, classical, Germanic and Christian traditions (Conley, 2014). Gender is of significance, and this remained the case in the 15th and 16th centuries, where English statutes concerning SVA focused mainly on rape, which was considered theft of a man's property (Armstrong, Gleckman-Krut and Johnson, 2018). As such, often the woman's suffering was deemed irrelevant and emphasis was placed on male relatives, who were considered the real victims of the crime, given that rape was viewed as a property crime. Having said this, there is evidence that legislation did distinguish between forcible violence and consensual sex and in Talmudic, Roman and early Christian and Germanic sources. Here, it was necessary to prove that force had been used and that the victim had resisted, which presented significant challenges and often relied on evidence of injury and in cases where women submitted out of fear or incapacity were considered consensual (Conley, 2014), you can see the result of this in current practice with the rape myth assumption that survivors should have physical injuries etc. following an assault. During the 16th and 17th centuries, religious values amplified notions of immorality and focused very much on the sexual component of rape. At the time all sex outside marriage was considered an offence, and as such, the victims of sexual violence were usually deemed guilty (Conley, 2014).

Whilst legislation existed relating mainly to rape, it must be noted that the legal system was operated by men; the standards of proof were difficult to meet and with the chances of conviction being almost non-existent; many victims were unwilling to come forward, a trend that has not lifted. This means it is difficult to understand the true historical prevalence of SVA. D'Cruze (1993) provides an excellent discussion exploring the history of SVA both from a societal and cultural perspective. This is worth a read to gain an in-depth understanding of the true nature of sexual violence and how this historical outlook impacts current discourse surrounding the topic.

The Industrial Revolution and emerging dominance of the middle class and their values, which emphasised the preservation of women's chastity, served to embed male dominance. Effectively the restriction of and control of women's sexuality was in the power of men, not only via the judicial system but also by fathers and husbands who were legally entitled to assert their patriarchal dominance and women were expected to place themselves under their protection (D'Cruze, 1993). During this time, women who lost chastity were labelled and deemed to have fallen, regardless of circumstance. In the mid-19th century the number of reported cases and prosecutions rose rapidly, and it is suggested that this reflected social values of the time, where male chivalry and feminine delicacy were emphasised, alongside recognition of individual rights and increased policing activity (Conley, 2014). In 1861, the Offences Against the Person Act attempted to consolidate legislation, focusing on a range of sexual crimes against women (UK Parliament, 2022) but prosecutions remained difficult. The requirement for the victim to prove their innocence was an enduring feature of how SVA was managed and whilst this period saw an increase in reporting, this was not sustained, and the number of prosecutions declined following World War 1 and did not rise again until the 1970s.

Building on medical advances and legislation passed in the 1960s which allowed women to control their fertility, the 1970s witnessed significant social and cultural change, particularly in relation to women's rights and liberation. This has been referred to the second wave of feminism (the first occurring between the late 1800s and early 1900s when women fought for the right to vote and originating in developed countries, such as the UK and USA). During and following this second wave of feminist activism, there was heightened awareness of the wide-ranging inequalities experienced by women, and this resulted in significant legislative changes relating to the role of women in society, including but not exclusively in relation to equal pay, protection of rights for pregnant women, as well as establishing the rights of women in the UK to take legal action against their spouse in the presence of domestic violence and abuse (Binard, 2017). These changes were significant but contained many loopholes and limitations, for example, the failure of legislation to protect women from martial rape (introduced in 1991), and to extend to protect those who were not married. Equally, despite these developments, violence against women remaines widespread (Binard, 2017).

The Conservative and Liberal Democrat coalition government (2010–2015) acknowledged key figures published by the ONS, which showed that between 2012 and 2013 around 1.2 million women suffered domestic abuse and over 330,000 women were sexually assaulted in the UK (UK Government, 2015). Here, there was political recognition of the need to encourage reporting, and to support survivors in rebuilding their lives, ensuring perpetrators were brought to justice, and importantly do more to prevent violence of all forms against women and girls. With almost £40 million of funding a range of activities were introduced, including re-launching high-profile media campaigns, working with TV and media to raise awareness, alongside national roll out of the domestic violence disclosure scheme (Clare's Law) which enabled police to disclose information to the public about a partner's previous violent offending. There was also a review of the police response to domestic violence and initiation of a programme of preventative work around SVA (UK Government, 2015). Whilst many campaigns have been aimed at reducing VAWG, there is a clear disconnect between these campaigns and a reduction of SVA.

## The Current Situation

It is difficult to determine the extent to which SVA occurs, as many do not report it to the police, and therefore, it is suggested that the data only reveals the tip of the iceberg (EVAW, 2022b). According to the Office for National Statistics (ONS) (2021a,b), five in six women and four in five men who are raped do not report this to the police.

Recent data from Rape Crisis England and Wales (2022) suggests that 1 in 4 women have experienced SVA as an adult; 1 in 6 children have been sexually abused and 1 in 20 men have been raped or sexually assaulted as an adult. It is also reported that one in two adult survivors of SVA have experienced it more than once. One in two rapes against women are carried out by their partner and in five out of six rapes against women, the perpetrator is known to them; one in three adult survivors of rape experienced it in their own home. The latest ONS (2021) data shows that Black and mixed-race adults are more likely to experience SVA than white or Asian adults. Overall, 3.62% of reported cases are experienced by mixed-race women; 2.89% by Black adults, whereas 1.38% of cases are among Asian adults and 2.03% in white adults. Those with a disability are at higher risk and account for 5% of reported cases. According to EVAW (2022a), the data does not capture fully the experience of all adults, for example, older adults living in institutions, such as care homes are not captured.

Rape Crisis England and Wales (2022) refer to SVA as a pandemic, and rightly so. The number of sexual offences recorded by the police in the year ending June 2022 showed an increase of 21% compared to the data for the year ending March 2020 (ONS, 2022). Figures were lower during lockdown and have increased substantially since, as you can see from the previous chapter. Of all recorded sexual offences, 36% were rape offences (ONS, 2022). The latest figures are alarming and may reflect an increase in the number of people experiencing SVA but may also be a result of campaigns encouraging victims and survivors to report their experience to the police and the impact of high-profile cases reported in the media (ONS, 2022). Of concern, whilst the highest ever number of rapes recorded by the police occurred in the year ending March 2022, charges were brought in only 2,223 of rape cases, and 98% of these prosecutions were against male perpetrators. This reflects historical patterns of poor conviction rates mentioned previously and in the presence of higher rates and higher rates of reporting. Rape Crisis England and Wales (2022) suggest that convictions are at their lowest since records began.

It is also essential to recognise that SVA is not a crime targets to younger people. In a study by Lea, Hunt and Shaw (2011), 6% of SA cases were found to have been survivors of an older age group (over 65 years); they go on to suggest that this number is significantly underestimated and will gradually increase alongside an ever-ageing population. Nevertheless, only a small body of research explores this age group in relation to the topic. Bows and Westmarland's (2016) freedom of information (FOI) research from 45 UK police forces found that from 87,230 cases of reported rape and sexual assault by penetration, 0.75% of survivors were recorded as being 60+ years, which are lower rates compared with previous research (Jeary, 2005; Ball and Fowler, 2008; Lea, Hunt and Shaw, 2011). The ONS UK lifestyle survey has recently increased their age limit (for people to complete) from 59 years to 74 years. Omitting people aged older than 74 from statistical analysis provides an inaccurate picture regarding SVA in the UK and, in turn, minimises SVA prevalence in this age group. Much of the prevention guidance is also aimed at younger people, again dismissing the potential of providing tangible support to older people and, potentially, impacting the number of survivors willing to report to formal sources. Not recognising older adults on government surveys and information contributes to an assumption that their assault will not be taken seriously. Walby and Allen (2004) suggest that a contributing factor may be confusion regarding the nature of SVA perpetrated by partners (i.e., hidden rape and a lack of understanding as to the nature of consent and changes to laws regarding rape in marriage).

Bows and Westmarland (2016) state by omitting this age group, the government are surrendering to rape myth stereotypes in their approach to collecting data. They clearly state that bracketing SVA survivors as young implies that older people are asexual and fuel the ageist approach of sex being a taboo subject in society. It could be argued that this taboo makes it more difficult for a practitioner to approach the topic with this group of service users, potentially missing opportunities to support survivors. Lea, Hunt and Shaw (2011) further support this by suggesting family, friends and professionals may miss the signs of SA in older adults due to society's stereotyping.

It is important to be aware these only touch the surface of the real story of SVA in society. This is due to a range of factors which include as follows: under reporting, lack of adequate recording of incidences when they are disclosed, attrition rates of cases, disbelieving attitudes, cross-cultural beliefs of what SVA is, and exclusion of large pockets of the population in most studies or data collection methods. Consequently, it is impossible to accurately measure the prevalence of SVA amongst the population. As a result, statistics surrounding SVA are acknowledged to be vastly underestimated and, as such, should be interpreted with caution. Increased recording of these statistics is becoming more common, and, whilst this has begun to give a greater insight of the scale of all types of SVA globally, far more people experience incidences of SVA than will ever report it, with some estimations being at 83% not reporting worldwide (Ceelen et al., 2019; Home Office, 2022).

In recent years there has been increasing recognition in the UK of the widespread and enduring prevalence of SVA, and, whilst it is accepted that men and boys can also be victims, these crimes disproportionately affect women and girls (UK Government, 2022). The VAWG statement published by the UK Government in 2022 covers a range of unacceptable crimes, including rape and other sexual offences, stalking, domestic abuse, 'honour'-based abuse (includes female genital mutilation, forced marriage and so-called honour-killings), revenge porn and many other forms of VAWG. It is noted that these crimes produce deep distress and affect victims of all ages, abilities, sexualities and backgrounds. The VAWG statement builds on the National Statement of Expectations (NSE) published in 2016 (Home Office, 2016), which set out how local areas should commission services to respond to VAWG and focus both on prevention but also ensuring victims and survivors had access to the help they need. The NSE had a clear focus on perpetrators, ensuring they were brought to justice, but also that the risk they pose is managed in order to keep victims/potential victims safe. The NSE emphasised the role of all key services, including police, local authorities, the NHS and the specialist VAWG sector in bringing about systemic changes, and between 2021 and 2022 the government have pledged just under £151 million to support victim and witness support services and community-based SVA services. Whilst the Office for Health Improvement and Disparities (2023) does not specifically refer to SVA, their priority areas below are of key importance in understanding and addressing this significant public health issue:

- identify and address health disparities, focusing on those groups and areas where health inequalities have greatest effect.
- take action on the biggest preventable risk factors for ill health and premature death, including tobacco, obesity and harmful use of alcohol and drugs.
- work with the NHS and local government to improve access to the services which detect and act on health risks and conditions, as early as possible.
- develop strong partnerships across government, communities, industry and employers, to act on the wider factors that contribute to people's health, such as work, housing and education.
- drive innovation in health improvement, harnessing the best of technology, analytics and innovations in policy and delivery, to help deliver change where it is needed most.

Alongside increased funding, a raft of policy and legislation have been introduced in recent years, including but not exclusively, the Domestic Abuse Act (2021) which introduced new measures to strengthen protection for victims of domestic abuse, the introduction of a Domestic Abuse Commissioner for England and Wales and the New Domestic Abuse Statutory Guidance (NHS England, 2022).

Although it is too early to understand the impact of increased policy and funding, some of the measures have been criticised by the End Violence Against Women (EVAW)

Coalition. The coalition is a group of feminist organisations and experts from across the UK, including specialist women's support services, activists, researchers, survivors and non-governmental organisations, established in 2005, whose aim is to end VAWG in all its forms. Andrea Simon, Director of the End Violence Against Women Coalition (2022a), stated that whilst over the last year some of the reforms felt like government was listening, what has happened is a series of superficial and short-sighted measures narrowly focused on keeping women safe on the streets via the introduction of street lighting, CCTV and increased police presence, compounded by changes to legislation that serve to deepen inequality for Black, minoritised, migrant and marginalised survivors of abuse via changes to the Policing Bill, the Nationality and Borders Bill and other legislative amendments. Simon suggests that what we need to see is properly funded transformational preventative work in schools, online safety laws and multi-year public campaigns to shift the attitudes that trivialise and normalise this abuse. Fundamentally, an approach to ending VAWG that focuses on safety is limited and what we need is a comprehensive, rights-based approach for all women (EVAW, 2022a).

### Who Carries Out Rape and Other Sexual Offences?

As mentioned previously, whilst it is known that some men are survivors of SVA, of those who are perpetrators and prosecuted, 98% are men. ONS (2021) data from the year ending December 2017 revealed that 10,317 men were prosecuted for sexual offences. Of these, 826 were aged 18–20; 1,100 were aged 21–24 and 8,391 were 25 and above. These numbers compare to only 177 women who were prosecuted in the same year for sexual offences. Of these, 17 were aged 18–20; 30 were 21–24 years of age and 130 were over 25 years of age (ONS, 2021).

Recent data from the Independent Office for Police Conduct (2021) highlights there has been a sharp increase in the number of disciplinary proceedings against police officers who abuse their position for a sexual purpose. Based on this and other sources of data, the EVAW Commission (2022b) notes that over 750 Metropolitan police employees have faced allegations of sexual misconduct since 2010, with only 83 being dismissed, one woman a week reports domestic abuse by a police officer and around 2,000 officers have faced accusations of sexual wrongdoing since 2017. Again, over 60% of these cases did not result in disciplinary action and only 8% were dismissed. The significance of this is that it illustrates the extent of sexism and misogyny in society but also produces a culture of mistrust of those in power and authority and further barriers to those at risk or who have experienced SVA seeking help and support (EVAW, 2022a). It is important to consider that if this resides within the police, it could also be replicated in other public organisations. There is very little data exploring the culture of SVA within the NHS; however, considering the systematic abuse captured within other large organisations, this is an area that desperately needs further exploration to ensure service users (and staff) are safeguarded and protected against risk of possible SVA and coercive power misuse.

### Disclosure

SVA disclosures have increased risks to the survivors who are highly complex, specifically when considering the statistics explored above, that the majority of survivors know their perpetrator, and the personal nature of the assault. Consequently, it often results in implications for the survivor's life and family following the disclosure. Ullman (2011) found disclosure of SVA was ultimately helpful to survivors, however, as this is mostly dependent on the response of the recipient.

Most research finds that disclosure (approximately 60–80%) will often be to a friend or family member (Dunn, Vail-Smith and Knight, 1999; Fisher et al., 2003; Ahrens et al., 2007; Ullman, 2010; Ullman and Peter-Hagene, 2014). Golding et al. (1989) and Koss et al. (1988) found similar results in their retrospective studies; that approximately two-thirds of complainants tell someone at some point but do not always seek professional support. Current statistics surrounding SVA are significantly underestimated due to lack of disclosure. Of those who experience SVA and do disclose, it is suggested that approximately 5–34% will disclose the SVA to a formal source such as healthcare professionals, police, psychologist and clergy (Starzynski and Ullman, 2014; Orchowski and Gidycz, 2015).

As the number of reported incidents of SVA has begun to increase, so does the likelihood of healthcare professionals experiencing disclosure within the healthcare setting and/or caring for an individual who may have experienced SVA but is yet to disclose. HCPs' roles are continually evolving, leading to an increase in responsibility (particularly with advanced clinical management), and this means that they are significantly more likely to receive and support disclosures of SVA. Disclosures or indicators of SVA could be identified within any area of health and social care where a therapeutic relationship has been established or built, whether in an acute or community setting. When considering the number of potential survivors identified above, the implications of disclosure on health and well-being, from both the survivor's perspective and for health and social services, are considerable. Chapter 3 focuses much more in depth on disclosure.

## The Impact on the Individual

The impact of SVA is not fully understood due to it largely being a hidden crime, often with no obvious identified indicators that are specific to these crimes. People who have experienced SVA often present in different ways depending on demographics and gender; however, the commonality of all is having had and continuing to have experienced serious complex trauma. Feelings of profound fear, terror and anxiety have been described by survivors, with safety and trust being significant factors that will continue to impact their life, in all ways. It is also wide known that the damage and devastation are enormous, extremely varied and often lifelong. SVA-associated post-traumatic stress (PTS) is a significant public health concern due to the substantial ongoing health implications for the survivor. These include (but are not limited to) as follows: anxiety, stress, fear, nervousness, social isolation, flashbacks, sleeping difficulties, drug/alcohol reliance, low self-esteem, increased cancer risks, self-harm and suicide. Understanding what happens before, during and after disclosure will provide greater insight on the support needed to improve health outcomes. This is explored further in Chapter 10.

## Social Cost

Whilst it is difficult to determine the true social cost of SVA, a study by Heeks et al. (2018) reported on the economic costs of crime for the Home Office. They found that of all non-fatal crimes, SVA (rape, specifically) had the highest estimated social cost at £39,360 per offence, which accounted to a total cost of £4.8 billion for the year based on an estimated number of 121,746 offences; other sexual offences were at £7.4 billion. The costs were attributed to managing the physical and emotional harm experienced by survivors, as well as the costs associated with time away from work and the associated costs for preventative measures. So, here, whilst this crime has the highest societal cost, alongside the high cost to the individual, it is concerning that this crime has one of the lowest prosecution rates, and the gap between rapes, their reports and prosecutions continues to widen (Hermolle, Andrews and Huang, 2022). Importantly, there is great variation across England and Wales. Home Office (2022) data show that Durham is the best performing area, where survivors are ten times more likely to see their case result in a charge than the worst performing area, Wiltshire. In Durham, 7.1% of rapes result in a charge compared to 0.7% in Wiltshire, 1.1% in Kent, 1.9% in Greater Manchester. The prosecution rates are alarmingly low and are falling. Overall, 41% of rape survivors withdraw their support for action and in London 65% withdrew support, rising by 7% from the previous year (EVAW, 2022a).

## Consent

If your role puts you in a position whereby you may receive disclosures of SVA, it is important to understand what is often defined as consent. Consent in the context of SVA refers to the voluntary and informed agreement between all parties involved in a sexual activity. It is an essential aspect of healthy and respectful sexual contact. Consent means that all individuals involved in a sexual encounter willingly agree to participate, and they have the capacity to make that decision freely. Here are some key principles and aspects of consent in the context of SVA:

**Voluntary:** Consent must be given willingly and without any form of pressure, coercion or manipulation. It should not be assumed or taken for granted.

**Informed:** All parties should have a clear understanding of what they are agreeing to. This includes understanding the nature of the sexual activity, potential risks and the ability to communicate boundaries and limits.

**Continuous:** Consent is not a one-time agreement. It should be ongoing and can be withdrawn at any point during the sexual encounter. If someone says 'no' or indicates discomfort or changes their mind, consent is no longer valid, and the activity should stop immediately.

**Freely given:** Consent cannot be obtained through intimidation, threats or any form of pressure. Both verbal and non-verbal cues should be respected. Silence or passivity should not be interpreted as consent.

**Capacity:** All parties involved should have the mental and emotional capacity to give consent. This means they should be of legal age and not under the influence of drugs or alcohol that impair their judgement.

**Equality:** Consent should be given by individuals on equal footing. Power imbalances, such as those based on age, authority or status, should not be exploited.

**Clear communication:** It is important for individuals to communicate their boundaries, desires and limits clearly. Effective communication helps ensure that all parties are on the same page.

**Respect for boundaries:** Respecting and honouring each person's boundaries is a fundamental aspect of sexual consent. Consent does not give anyone the right to disregard another person's limits.

**Revocable:** Consent can be revoked at any time. If someone decides they are no longer comfortable with the sexual activity, their decision to stop should be respected immediately.

**Understanding non-verbal cues:** Paying attention to non-verbal cues, such as body language and facial expressions, is crucial for understanding whether someone is comfortable with the ongoing sexual activity.

Consent is an ongoing process and should be sought and confirmed throughout any sexual encounter. It is the responsibility of all parties involved to ensure that they have received clear and enthusiastic consent before proceeding with any sexual activity. Failure to obtain proper consent can lead to serious ethical and legal consequences, including sexual assault charges. It is essential, as HCPs, we educate service users to prioritise open communication, respect and empathy when it comes to sexual health and relationships.

## Summary of the Chapter

This chapter has introduced SVA highlighting key definitions and terminology. The chapter has considered what we know about who perpetrates SVA, as well as some of what is known about those who have experienced it. In doing this, the chapter has included some historical context, as well as introducing some of the contemporary approaches to understanding and addressing SVA.

## References

Ahrens, C. E., Campbell, R., Ternier-Themes, N., Wasco, S. M. and Sefl, T. (2007) 'Deciding whom to tell: expectations and outcomes of rape survivors' first disclosures', *Psychology of Women's Quarterly*, 31, pp. 38–49.

Armstrong, E. A., Gleckman-Krut, M. and Johnson, L. (2018) 'Silence, power and inequality: An intersectional approach to sexual violence', *Annual Review of Sociology*, 44(1), pp. 99–122. https://doi.org/10.1146/annurev-soc-073117-041410

Ball, H. N. and Fowler, D. (2008) 'Sexual offending against older female victims: An empirical study of the prevalence and characteristics of recorded offences in a semi-rural English county', *Journal of Forensic Psychiatry & Psychology*, 19(1), pp. 14–32.

Binard, F. (2017) 'The British women's liberation movement in the 1970s: Redefining the personal and the political', *French Journal of British Studies*. Online since 30 December 2017. http://journals.openedition.org/rfcb/1688; https://doi.org/10.4000/rfcb.1688

Bows, H. and Westmarland, N. (2016) 'Rape of older people in the United Kingdom challenging the 'real-rape' stereotype', *British Journal of Criminology*, 57(1), pp. 1–17.

Ceelen, M., Dorn, T., Flora, S. and van Huisand Reijnders, U. J. L. (2019) 'Characteristics and post-decision attitudes of non-reporting sexual violence Victims', *Journal of Interpersonal Violence*, 34(9), pp. 1961–1977.

Conley, A. C. (2014). "Chapter 12: Sexual Violence in Historical Perspective". In Gartner, R. and McCarthy, B. (Eds.), *The Oxford Handbook of Gender, Sex and Crime* (pp. 207–224). Oxford: Oxford University Press Online.

Crime Survey of England and Wales (CSEW) (2021) The Crime Survey for England and Wales. Available at: https://www.ons.gov.uk/peoplepopulationandcommunity/crimeandjustice/bulletins/crimeinenglandandwales/yearendingseptember2021

D'Cruze, S. (1993) 'Approaching the history of rape and sexual violence: Notes towards research', *Women's History Review*, 1(3), pp. 377–397.

Domestic Abuse Act (2021) Available at: https://www.legislation.gov.uk/ukpga/2021/17/contents/enacted

Dunn, P. C., Vail-Smith, K. and Knight, S. M. (1999) 'What date/acquaintance rape victims tell others: A study of college student recipients of disclosure', *Journal of American College Health*, 47(5), pp. 213–219. https://doi.org/10.1080/07448489909595650

End Violence Against Women (EVAW) (2022a) Violence Against Women and Girls. Snapshot Report 2021–22. Available at: https://www.endviolenceagainstwomen.org.uk/wp-content/uploads/EVAW-snapshot-report-FINAL-030322.pdf

End Violence against Women (EVAW) (2022b) Latest Data Shows More Sexual Offences Recorded Than Ever Before. Available at: https://www.endviolenceagainstwomen.org.uk/latest-data-shows-more-sexual-offences-recorded-than-ever-before/

Fisher, B. S., Daigle, L. E., Cullen, F. T. and Turner, M. G. (2003) 'Reporting sexual victimization to the police and others: Results from a national-level study of college women', *Criminal Justice Behaviour*, 30(1), pp. 6–38.

Golding, J. M., Siege, J. M., Sorenson, S. B., Burnam, A. M. and Stein, J. (1989) 'Social support sources following sexual Assault', *Journal of Community Psychology*, 17(1), pp. 92–107.

Guerette, S. M. and Caron, S. L. (2007) 'Assessing the impact of acquaintance rape: Interviews with women who are victims/survivors of sexual assault while in college', *Journal of College Student Psychotherapy*, 22(2), pp. 31–50.

Heeks, M., Reed, S., Tasfiri, M. and Prince, S. (2018) *The Economic and Social Costs of Crime*. London: Home Office.

Hermolle, M., Andrews, S. J. and Huang, C.-Y. S. (2022) 'Race stereotype acceptance in the general population of England and Wales', *Journal of Interpersonal Violence*. Online First. https://doi.org/10.1177/08862605221076162

Hockett, J. M. and Saucier, D. A. (2015) 'A systematic literature review of "rape victims" versus "rape survivors": Implications for theory, research, and practice', *Aggression and Violent Behaviour*, 25, pp. 1–14. https://doi.org/10.1016/j.avb.2015.07.003

Holstein, J. A. and Miller, G. (1990) 'Rethinking victimisation: An international approach to victimology', *Symbolic Interaction*, 13(1), pp. 103–122.

Home Office (2016) Violence Against Women and Girls. National Statement of Expectations. Available at: https://assets.publishing.service.gov.uk/government/uploads/system/uploads/attachment_data/file/574665/VAWG_National_Statement_of_Expectations_-_FINAL.PDF

Home Office (2022) Crime Outcomes in England and Wales 2021 to 2022. Available at: https://www.gov.uk/government/statistics/crime-outcomes-in-england-and-wales-2021-to-2022/crime-outcomes-in-england-and-wales-2021-to-2022

Horvath, M. and Brown, J. (Eds.) (2022) *Rape; Challenging Contemporary Thinking*. New York, NY: Routledge.

Independent Office for Police Conduct (2021) There Must Be Nowhere to Hide for Police Who Abuse Their Position for a Sexual Purpose. Available at: https://www.policeconduct.gov.uk/news/there-must-be-nowhere-hide-police-who-abuse-their-position-sexual-purpose

Jeary, K. (2005) 'Sexual abuse and sexual offending against elderly people: A focus on perpetrators and victims', *Journal of Forensic Psychiatry and Psychology*, 16(2), pp. 328–343.

Koss, M. P., Dinero, T. E., Seibel, C. A. and Cox, S. L. (1988) 'Stranger and acquaintance rape: Are there differences in the victim's experience?', *Psychology of Women Quarterly*, 12(1), pp. 1–24.

Lea, S. J., Hunt, L. and Shaw, S. (2011) 'Sexual assault of older women by strangers', *Journal of Interpersonal Violence*, 26(11), pp. 2303–2320.

Lois, F. H. (2021) Sexual Assault As a Weapon of War: History and Prevention. Available at: https://medium.com/ngwomen4peace/sexual-assault-as-a-weapon-of-war-history-and-prevention-72cf9c73e090

Ministry of Justice (2022) Support for Victims of Sexual Violence and Abuse. Available at: https://www.gov.uk/guidance/support-for-victims-of-sexual-violence-and-abuse#what-is-sexual-violence-and-abuse

NHS England (2022) Strategic Direction for Sexual Assault and Abuse Services. Lifelong Care for Victims and Survivors: 2018–2023. Available at: https://www.england.nhs.uk/wp-content/uploads/2018/04/strategic-direction-sexual-assault-and-abuse-services.pdf

Office for Health Improvement and Disparities. About Us. Available at: https://www.gov.uk/government/organisations/office-for-health-improvement-and-disparities/about#priorities

Office for National Statistics (ONS) (2021a) Sexual Offences in England and Wales Overview: Year Ending March 2020. Available at: https://www.ons.gov.uk/peoplepopulationandcommunity/crimeandjustice/bulletins/sexualoffencesinenglandandwalesoverview/march2020

Office for National Statistics (ONS) (2021b) Crime Survey for England and Wales. Available at: https://www.ons.gov.uk/peoplepopulationandcommunity/crimeandjustice/bulletins/crimein englandandwales/yearendingmarch2022#:~:text=Police%20recorded%20crime%20in%20 England,2020%20(6.1%20million%20offences)

Office for National Statistics (ONS) (2022) Crime in England and Wales: Year Ending June 2022. https://www.ons.gov.uk/peoplepopulationandcommunity/crimeandjustice/bulletins/crimeinenglandandwales/yearendingjune2022#domestic-abuse-and-sexual-offences

Orchowski, L. M. and Gidycz, C. A. (2015) 'Psychological consequences associated with positive and negative responses to disclosure of sexual assault among college women: A prospective Study', *Violence Against Women*, 21(7), pp. 803–823.

Parker, J. A. and Mahlstedt, D. (2010) 'Language, Power, and Sexual Assault: Women's Voices on Rape and Social Change'. In Behrens, S. J. and Parker, J. (Eds.), *Language in the Real World: An Introduction to Linguistics*. New York, NY: Routledge.

Patterson, D. and Campbell, R. (2010) 'Why rape survivors participate in the criminal justice system', *Journal of Community Psychology*, 38(3), pp. 191–205.

Rape Crisis England and Wales (2022) Statistics About Sexual Violence and Abuse. Available at: https://rapecrisis.org.uk/get-informed/statistics-sexual-violence/

Sexual Offences Act (2003) Sexual Offences Act 2003. Available at: https://www.legislation.gov.uk/ukpga/2003/42/contents

Starzynski, L. L. and Ullman, S. E. (2014) 'Correlates of perceived helpfulness of mental health professionals following disclosure of sexual assault', *Violence Against Women*, 20(1), pp. 74–94.

The Survivors Trust (2022) Men Overcoming Sexual Violence Together. Available at: https://www.survivorsuk.org/about-us/#section-1

Thompson, M. (2000) 'Life after rape: A chance to speak', *Sexual and Relationship Therapy*, 15(4), pp. 325–343.

UK Government (2015) 2010–2015 Government Policy: Violence Against Women and Girls. Available at: https://www.gov.uk/government/publications/2010-to-2015-government-policy-violence-against-women-and-girls/2010-to-2015-government-policy-violence-against-women-and-girls

UK Government (2022) Violence Against Women and Girls National Statement of Expectations. Available at: https://www.gov.uk/government/publications/violence-againstwomen-and-girls-national-statement-of-expectations-and-commissioning-toolkit/violence-against-women-and-girls-national-statement-of-expectations-accessible

UK Parliament (2022) Regulating Sexual Behaviour: The 19th Century. Available at: https://www.parliament.uk/about/living-heritage/transformingsociety/private-lives/relationships/overview/sexualbehaviour19thcentury/

Ullman, S. E. (2011) 'Is disclosure of sexual traumas helpful? Comparing experimental laboratory verses field study results', *Journal of Aggression, Maltreatment and Trauma*, 20(2), pp. 148–162.

Ullman, S. E. (2010) *Talking About Sexual Assault: Society's Response to Survivors*. Washington, DC: American Psychological Association. https://doi.org/10.1037/12083-000

Ullman, S. E. and Peter-Hagene, L. (2014) 'Social reactions to sexual assault disclosure, coping, perceived control, and PTSD symptoms in sexual assault victims', *Journal of Community Psychology*, 42(4), pp. 495–508.

Walby, S. and Allen, J. (2004). *Domestic violence, sexual assault and stalking: findings from the British Crime Survey*. London: Home Office

# 3    Disclosures of Sexual Violence and Abuse

## Introduction

This chapter considers how sexual violence and abuse (SVA) is often come across in practice, with particular emphasis on disclosure, barriers to disclosure and the implications of this for the individual and for healthcare practitioners (HCP).

## Disclosure

Disclosure of SVA refers to telling (in any form) another person(s) about that experience. SVA is a traumatic life event and, whilst disclosing trauma has long been associated with positive effects (Pennebaker, 1997), the application of this to sexual trauma has often led to inconsistent findings (Ullman, Foynes and Tang, 2010). SVA disclosures have increased risks to the survivors, who are highly complex, especially when considering 90% of survivors know their perpetrator, and because of the personal nature of the assault. Understanding the complexities of disclosure will have a positive impact on your service user, although it is essential to remember that disclosure often results in implications for the survivor's life following the disclosure (for example, relationship breakdown). Ullman (2011) found that disclosure of trauma is useful from the perspective of seeking tangible support; however, from an SVA perspective, more exploration of the positive and negative implications (on the survivor) of disclosing trauma in healthcare is required to better understand the support people may need, to avoid negative responses, and facilitate supportive disclosures.

People who do not seek support following an experience of SVA are at risk of depression and post-traumatic stress (PTS); however, it is also worth noting that those who disclose and receive negative reactions from their healthcare provider (or anyone) often have higher levels of depression, PTS and ongoing physical and mental health problems (Ahrens, Stansell and Jennings, 2010). This strengthens the need for healthcare practitioners to be adequately prepared to support disclosures.

## Barriers to Disclosure

Since the 1970s, researchers and feminist activists have been increasingly exploring the dynamics that keep survivors from speaking about their experiences of SVA. Feminist literature argues that the active function of powerlessness is a main reason for women not disclosing, and that silencing women serves to reinforce powerlessness (Brownmiller, 1976; Koss, 1985; MacKinnon, 1994; Abby, McAuslan and Ross, 1998). As a societal concept, powerlessness applies to formal sources where disclosure may determine a wider

DOI: 10.4324/9781003225461-3

range of repercussions, meaning silencing is caused by many factors (fear of blame, fear of the SVA being reported to the police without permission, fear of not being able to control what happens after disclosure and shame. Accessing healthcare often results in a power imbalance; feeling unsupported in disclosing may silence survivors to refrain from further disclosure, seeking further support, and potentially, reporting their assault to the authorities.

Patterson, Greeson and Campbell (2009) found that women identify multiple reasons for not accessing any support (feelings of self-blame, shame and anticipated rejection) that, ultimately, made them not want to share their experience. Self-blame and shame were related to rape myths associated with stereotypical (stranger, violence) and non-stereotypical (offender known and non-violence) rape experiences. Alongside this is the belief that women were self-protecting themselves from harm (not being believed, feeling vulnerable, being probed with questions that would relive the trauma and not wanting to be touched). This is insightful as it emphasises the need for healthcare practitioners to understand why survivors do not come forward to disclose and how we can ensure their experience is removed from these barriers. SVA is an experience that is loaded in societal misconceptions, often based on rape myths and victim-blaming assumptions; the impacts of these continue to hinder survivors from seeking support.

### Myths

Rape myths and victim-blaming assumptions have been identified as directly correlating with barriers to disclosure. Rape myths can be defined as stereotyped or false beliefs about rape, rape victims and rapists (Burt, 1980). Rape myths influence and reinforce (from a societal perspective) what is, and is not SVA, as well as who are, and who are not, deemed credible victims of rape. This has implications for victims, offenders and societal assumptions in the way survivors of SVA are (or are not) supported following disclosure. Lonsway and Fitzgerald (1994) describe this as attitudes and beliefs that are generally untrue but are widely and persistently believed.

Rape myths directly contribute to victim-blaming behaviours, and this behaviour overtly places the blame of the assault on the survivor. Victim blaming can be defined as someone implying or treating a person who has experienced SVA as if it was a result of something they did or said, instead of placing the responsibility where it belongs: on the person who harmed them. Examples of these can be found in Table 3.1.

Ullman and Filipas (2001) suggest that women do not always report rape because they often perceive that they are at fault themselves. Starzynski et al. (2005) suggest that as a society we have a preconceived, socially constructed mindset that SVA is violent, that those being attacked will fight back, that it is anonymous and life threatening. However, it is frequently the opposite: the attacker often being a romantic partner, family member, friend or acquaintance (in more than 90% of experiences). The survivor often freezes, as not to anger their attacker further, and, more often, the actual rape is not life threatening (McCabe and Wauchope, 2005). Intimate partner or acquaintance assaults are often more violent than stranger attacks, thereby diminishing the rape myths often adhered to regarding stranger rapes being more violent (Möller et al., 2012; Du Mont et al., 2017). This is important since those with violent experiences of SVA are more likely to access health services (Logan, Cole and Capillo, 2007; Möller et al., 2012); therefore, when you work in healthcare, it may be that your myth assumption supports this view as it is what you see most. Those who experience SVA within

*Table 3.1* Example of Rape Myths

| Myth | Fact |
|---|---|
| Women who drink or take drugs deserve it if they get raped. | No one is ever to blame for being raped or sexually assaulted. Overall, 100% of the blame, shame and responsibility for such crimes lie with the perpetrator. |
| Women lie about being raped for attention or if they regret having had sex with someone. | False allegations of rape are extremely rare. Most people who experience any form of sexual violence or abuse never tell the police. |
| If she didn't scream, try to run away or fight back, then it wasn't rape. | The body has an automatic response to fear, which is designed to protect us, and therefore, it is common for those who experience SVA (sexual violence and abuse) to find they can't move or speak. This explains why lots of people who have experienced SVA do not have visible injuries. |
| If they didn't say no, then it wasn't rape. | Not saying no is not consent. If someone seems unsure, is quiet, moves away or does not respond, they are not providing consent. |
| It is not rape if it is your partner. | Rape is always rape. If the person does not consent, regardless of relationship status. |
| Women are asking for it if they wear revealing clothes or flirt. | Women and girls, as with everyone, have the right to wear what they want and behave how they wish. There is never an excuse for rape or sexual assault. |
| Once a man is turned on, he can't help himself, he has to have sex. | There is no scientific basis in this myth and men can control themselves and should. Rape and all forms of SVA are serious crimes. |
| Women say no, when they really mean yes. | If someone says no, this should always be respected. Everyone has the right to change their minds at any point during sexual activity. |
| Survivors should act a certain way after being raped or experiencing SVA. | No, everyone responds differently. Some people do not feel the effects of trauma until a long time after the traumatic event has occurred. |

intimate relationships are less likely to report their assaults; HCPs need to be aware of this, in assessing risks whilst undertaking health assessments/histories. These survivors could be lost due to rape myths minimising the likelihood of the HCP asking more detailed questions about their health/sexual health/intimate injuries (Murphy et al., 2011; Möller et al., 2012).

Rape myth acceptance is often strongly associated with all types of prejudicial beliefs such as racism, homophobia, sexism, ageism (Suarez and Gadalla, 2010). It is clear that these barriers are not easing and are significantly impacting SVA disclosure, demonstrating a need for HCPs to receive education around SVA and to address and understand the intersectionality of oppressive belief systems.

There are many myths concerning SVA, Rape Crisis England and Wales (2022) and other organisations, work hard to dispel these and to present the facts. It is accepted that myths are culturally bound and cause serious harm both in terms of how survivors feel, the likelihood of them reporting their experience and seeking help, but also how survivors are treated by their friends, families and communities, as well as organisations and services.

Some of the key myths and facts are shown in Table 3.1 (Rape Crisis England and Wales, 2022).

According to Rape Crisis England and Wales (2022), such myths are a central feature of what is referred to as 'rape culture'. It is suggested that the term 'rape culture' was first used in a 1975 documentary entitled *Rape Culture* by Lazarus and Wunderlich, which used the term to describe the ways in which women's sexuality is commodified, their sexual agency minimised, whilst at the same time celebrating male dominance over women and ideals of violent masculinity (Peter and Besley, 2019). Whilst this term emerged in the USA, a similar term 'lad culture' has been used to refer to the objectification of women, normalisation of misogynist language and behaviours (Lewis, Marine and Kenney, 2016). Rape culture and the everyday sexism women face are thought to explain why the criminal justice system fails to hold perpetrators to account, but also why more has not been done to prevent and support victims and survivors (Rape Crisis England and Wales, 2022).

## Hidden Rape

Lack of acknowledgement of the experience as a form of SVA is another barrier to disclosure. Hidden rape is a concept whereby people who described having unwanted sex did not believe they had been raped (Koss 1989). Hidden rape is still common in society today and contributes to the unintended effect of reinforcing society's view of what constitutes SVA (Lanthier, Du Mont and Mason, 2018). Another term used to describe this is unacknowledged rape. Unacknowledged rape occurs when the survivor does not deem the assault as rape, but instead gives it a gentler label, such as 'miscommunication' (Littleton and Breitkopf, 2006), and thus ultimately hides or turns away from their experience. This is often the case when the perpetrator is known to the survivors, as survivors often feel they have a greater legitimacy if their experience was with stranger and have physical injuries to provide validation of experience, therefore aiding them to seek formal support (Starzynski and Ullman, 2014; McQueen et al., 2021). Survivors with 'classic' assault experience scenarios are more likely to report to the police, confirming that stereotypical assumptions of what constitutes SVA may affect disclosure (Ahrens, Stansell and Jennings 2010).

## Screening for SVA

Another identified barrier of disclosure in the healthcare setting is lack of screening for SVA experiences. Vandenberghe et al. (2018) suggest that healthcare staff indicate that they had insufficient knowledge regarding the prevalence of SVA. However, over half felt happy exploring experiences of SVA when they suspected it within their consultations. A general consistency among practitioners highlighted that asking about abuse had the potential to take them deep into a conversation that could be fraught with risk to both patients and them (Williston and Lafreniere, 2013). From the patient support perspective, opening a topic that the HCP has no knowledge or experience on, therefore, could potentially put the survivor at risk of not receiving adequate support. This also has impacts on the HCPs, for example, especially if they had previously experienced SVA personally, but also from the perspective of feeling lacking in the care they give due to limited knowledge.

Research findings throughout the past 30 years are consistent with low screening rates for SVA. Friedman et al. (1992) found that 6% of patients who attended private and public primary care settings (in the USA) had been asked if they had experienced SVA by physicians. Littleton, Berenson and Breitkopf (2007) highlighted a higher proportion, with 37% of women having been asked about SVA experiences. Berry and Rutledge (2016) found similarly that most participants (female) had never been screened for SVA (71.3%) by any healthcare provider they had accessed. Worryingly, this suggests that over the past three decades never more than one third of people are screened for SVA in healthcare practice, therefore potentially reducing signposting opportunities and subsequent access to support services and, in turn, increasing the likelihood of non-disclosure PTS.

Berry and Rutledge (2016) explored the factors that influenced women disclosing SVA to HCPs in primary care and found that women desired to be screened for SVA since this gave them a sense of permission to disclose. This therefore demonstrates the importance of screening for SVA, rather than making case-by-case decisions, based on symptoms which triggers HCPs to ask, which is the norm in most healthcare settings (e.g., looking for indicators). We need to remember that on the whole, women are not offended to be asked about experiences of SVA.

With the prevalence of SVA being at its highest (Home Office, 2022), HCPs are likely to care for survivors of SVA daily (World Health Organisation, 2013). As we have already identified, more than 50% of SVA survivors will go on to develop psychological responses with a large proportion being more likely to report physical symptoms, including chronic pain and health conditions, resulting from negative health behaviours such as increased alcohol and drug intake, smoking and eating disorders, unwanted pregnancies and risks of sexually transmitted infections (STIs). Littleton et al. (2007) highlighted 52% of women reporting that an HCP had never screened them or provided any sort of information regarding SVA. This lack of screening is also identified by McLindon and Harms (2011); they found 95% of nurses from a mental health unit believed SVA should not be explored so as not to increase the risk of trauma. Interestingly, fewer than 6% of women reported that they would find being screened for SVA history to be bothersome or upsetting, and more than 95% of women who received any of the types of information about SVA from a healthcare practitioner reported that this information was potentially helpful (Littleton, Berenson and Breitkopf, 2007). This discussion is important as it highlights that woman are not offended to be asked about their SVA history, contrary to HCP's perceived barriers. This opens a bigger discussion into perceived barriers of screening for SVA in clinical practice, as ultimately it shows that HCP's discussing SVA with their patients is a conversation most individuals are open to and can benefit from. That said, the response and support given to survivors of SVA must be received in a positive way to provide positive outcomes.

This highlights the need for HCPs to screen for SVA using a direct enquiry to their approach.

## Blame

Reactions to SVA disclosures contribute to whether, and how, survivors blame themselves for the SVA (Ullman and Najdowski, 2011). Sigurvinsdottir and Ullman (2015) explored social reactions (friends and family) in relation to post-disclosure self-blame and problem drinking in survivors. They found that negative reactions to SVA disclosure reinforced any self-blame survivors might have had and can lead to problem drinking and a lack of engagement with disclosing the assault to formal avenues, such as HCPs. Blame is typically one of the most harmful reactions that survivors will experience when disclosing SVA. Therefore, the concepts of self-blame must be understood by HCPs supporting survivors. Self-blame is consistent with adherence to victim-blaming attitudes. Survivors indicated that they were less likely to continue to disclose if they were met with rape myth assumptions, such as blame (Dworkin and Allen, 2018). It is clear that rape myths and victim-blaming assumptions largely contribute to SVA disclosure barriers and have done so for many years. Negative responses towards SVA disclosures are more common from formal support providers than from informal support providers, and the most common reaction from both police and HCPs was to blame the survivor, and this has been found over the past 22 years consistently, demonstrating the need for HCPs to critically explore our adherence to blame culture/myth adherence (Ullman, 1996; Filipas and Ullman, 2001; Ahrens et al., 2007; McQueen et al., 2021).

**Diversity and Disclosure**

Diversity is also acknowledged as playing a role in disclosure barriers (Washington, 2001; Tillman et al., 2010; Lindquist et al., 2016; Hakimi et al., 2018). Several cultural barriers have been identified, including distrust and avoidance of police, legal, medical, and social organisations (Lindquist et al., 2016), and family shame (Huong, 2012). There is a body of research that indicates that minoritised women are less likely to report an SVA than white women (Fisher et al., 2003; Krebs et al., 2011; Lindquist et al., 2016). However, overall, the barriers to reporting are similar across all cultural differences for the last 30 years: such as fear of not being believed, the use of drugs and alcohol prior to the assault, and lack of certainty that the experience was rape (Koss et al., 1988; Hakimi et al., 2018), with the consistent main addition being distrust in public officials (Washington, 2001; Hakimi et al., 2018). The reduction in disclosure linked to distrust in public officials is a constant that has not changed in over 20 years. Jacques-Tiura et al. (2010) explored experiences of SVA in both African American (52%) and Caucasian women (67%), accessing 272 participants who were currently not engaged in education. They found African American women described receiving more negative responses to their disclosure and higher levels of self-reported PTS following disclosure (Jacques-Tiura et al., 2010). Hakimi et al. (2018) also demonstrated that high negative reactions to Black women's disclosure resulted in higher levels of PTS than in white females, specifically around their finding of a main barrier being 'black women are strong and just need to get on with it'. Similarly, Huong (2012) explored the social support of rape in kin groups in Vietnam and found that disclosure is often bound to complexities of family honour and shame. In her study she found women's rape narratives are often pulled apart by other women in the community, with a focus on what the outcome would be for the perpetrator and his family. These types of beliefs and behaviours have been, and continue to be, mirrored in many marginalised patriarchal communities throughout the world (Heise, 1993; Hetu, 2020). This demonstrates that attitudes and perceptions are directly causing barriers to women from diverse backgrounds in accessing ongoing help and support.

Survivors from ethnically diverse backgrounds (for example, Asian, Latinas, indigenous or travelling communities), who do not/cannot access education, and those who fall outside of college/university age range (typically over 25-year-olds), are being left behind when it comes to understanding their disclosure experiences. In the UK and the USA there is also an increasing mistrust in formal support providers, such as the police, particularly from gender and racial perspectives (Johnson, Devereux and Wagner, 2022). These factors may deter people from accessing healthcare and other services, thus reducing the desire or opportunity for those disclosing to formal sources. This indicates that as HCPs we must consider these impacts when undertaking any form of SVA screening among marginalised groups.

## Children and Disclosure

The reason a child does not disclose episodes of SVA is different from the reason an adult does not disclose (Bagley and King, 1990; Hollies, 1990; Wilson, 1994); yet, much of the SVA education and/or training provided to HCPs surrounding SVA is focused on child safeguarding. Studies show children may not disclose SVA for many contextualised reasons; these include failure to recognise abuse as a problem, therefore not understanding they are in need of support, normalisation of SVA, lack of vocabulary to describe SVA, lack of support (for example, not having anyone to talk to) and like in adults: fear of repercussions either for themselves or the perpetrator, shame, stigma, guilt and self-blame. Washington (2001) suggests that children are selective in who they tell about their experience. This is influenced by a deep-rooted fear of being revictimised and the potential of being ostracised, specifically when the assailant is known by family and friends. When considering that 90% of survivors know their attacker, this makes disclosure even more difficult. Although much research suggests that few children disclose sexual abuse, a study by the UK organisation National Society for the Prevention of Cruelty to Children (Allnock and Miller, 2019) over 80% had tried to tell someone about the abuse; however, they were dismissed, played down or ignored.

## Men and Disclosure

It has long been reported that men are less likely to disclose SVA than women, and those numbers are not changing (Isley, 1998; Sable et al., 2006; Allen, Ridgeway and Swan, 2015; Walfield, 2018). It is acknowledged that men have additional barriers to disclosing when compared with women. Allen, Ridgeway and Swan (2015) found shame, guilt and/or embarrassment, fear of retaliation and fear of not being believed as the top barriers. Additionally, men identified 'not wanting to be perceived as gay' as a top barrier, supporting the discussion regarding social stigma (and homophobia) regarding male SVA survivors. Of those men who do disclose, they are more likely to disclose historic child sex abuse than an experience of SVA in adulthood (Graham, 2006; Javid, 2017). There are multiple barriers to men disclosing SVA that are cloaked in rape myths and victim-blaming assumptions, including (but not limited to) men cannot be raped; real men can defend themselves; women cannot sexually assault men; male rape only happens in prisons; men who are raped by other men are homosexual; if a man gets an erection, he must have wanted it; gay and bisexual men deserve to be raped because they are immoral/promiscuous (Sable et al., 2006; Turchik and Edwards, 2012). Allen, Ridgeway and Swan (2015) found that male survivors' barriers were focused on shame, guilt and embarrassment, not wanting friends or family to know, and services being aimed predominantly at females who have experienced SVA. A recent study (Walfield, 2018) indicated that most individuals adhere to male rape myths to some degree, demonstrating that male rape is also a hidden crime due to adherence in these beliefs. Often discussions and education surrounding SVA are largely framed in women's issues or women's services, and it could be argued that a preventative programme focusing on (self-) prevention for women, and consent classes for men, does not help to reduce the gender stereotypes. Therefore, norms of male rape should be challenged, for example, via societal approaches to sex and relationship education and consent classes focused on male and female experiences of SVA. Statistically, women are more at risk of SVA than men; however, as HCPs we must be aware that often the psychological support for men disclosing experiences may be different than women.

We acknowledge that there are people within society that have increased barriers to disclosure, on top of gender, age and ethnicity. This is addressed and explored further in Chapter 4.

## Survivors' Experiences of Disclosing to a Healthcare Practitioner

Ranjbar and Speer (2013) overwhelmingly reported negative experiences from survivors accessing healthcare for support following SVA, citing inexperience in dealing with survivors of SVA, disrespectful or inconsiderate treatment and HCPs adhering to myths and stereotypes surrounding SVA. The research does not state at which point in the service user's recovery these experiences occurred, although it highlighted the need for HCPs and their organisations to engage in education and/or training in the topic.

Due to the statistics, we have touched upon so far and the impact on psychological well-being (Khalifeh et al., 2011); it could be assumed that SVA should be high on the assessment agenda for those working in mental health facilities. However, evidence indicates that when disclosures of SVA are made by those with a diagnosed mental illness, they are often not made in plausible terms; therefore, it can be difficult to determine whether allegations are delusional episodes or not (Ashmore, Spangaro and McNamara, 2015). As a result, they are often minimised and, unfortunately, the minimisation of disclosures increases the likelihood of traumatic and aggressive reactions to negative responses from recipients, causing trust and communication barriers between survivors and HCPs (Ashmore, Spangaro and McNamara, 2015). McLindon and Harms (2011) found that over 95% of mental health practitioners participating in their study believed their patients should not be asked initially or further (should the service user have mentioned it) about sexual trauma, identifying increased risk of psychological distress as a reason to avoid the topic. Half of the sample expressed that they felt under confident in responding to disclosures. This is concerning, considering the estimated levels of those experiencing psychological trauma who have experienced SVA. Not addressing it would be of no advantage and, in some cases, detrimental to the survivor's ongoing health needs. It could also be suggested that not exploring this event at a time of crisis diminishes both the experience and the impact that experience has on the service user. Individuals should feel supported, and HCPs must emphasise the importance and safety of being able to disclose (Humphreys and Thiara, 2003). Concerningly, McLindon and Harms (2011) also found 73% of mental health staff highlighted that they had received no training or education in at least the last 10 years to enable them to confidently manage and discuss disclosures, with 60% stating that they used personal experience to guide their professional practice. Clearly this is a contributing factor to the discomfort some HCPs feel in addressing

SVA. Survivors can pick up this discomfort, for example, when considering an in-house recovery programme for substance abuse; Hunter, Robison and Jasin (2012) found that over 50% had disclosed their experiences of SVA to other residents. Therefore, in settings such as these, staff not only need to be aware of potentially responding to multiple PTS impacts of disclosure but also need to be aware of the impact of secondary trauma for those already in recovery.

HCPs are more likely to adhere to rape myth assumptions and not take disclosures seriously if survivors have mental health issues and/or are alcohol dependant (Ashmore, Spangaro and Mcnamara, 2015). This lack of support is mirrored by problem drinkers' social support mechanisms, highlighting that those with alcohol issues have decreased social and formal support, increasing the impact of their PTS which, in turn, results in worse health outcomes. Screening of SVA should be an essential component to HCPs' assessment and conversation, but only if the HCP is appropriately able to do so (with regard to education and/or training).

## Positive and Negative Outcomes of Disclosure

Positive and helpful attitudes of the HCP, together with increased comfort and trusting level, have been indicated as important for disclosure (Berry and Rutledge, 2016). One positive avenue for survivors is permission giving; this encourages disclosures to HCPs: validation and acknowledgement have been strongly attributed to positive experience as this gives the survivors a sense of being believed by the recipient (Ullman, 1996; Dunleavy and Slowik, 2012). Showing compassion and providing an empathetic response is consistently seen as providing positive emotional support (Ahrens, Cabral and Abeling, 2009; Ahrens, Stansell and Jennings 2010; Dunleavy and Slowik, 2012; Starzynski and Ullman, 2014; McQueen et al., 2021). This includes telling survivors that they were not to blame for the assault. Survivors' perception of helpfulness of HCPs suggests that positive outcomes are associated with empathy, emotional support and tangible aid, while similarly, not being believed is strongly linked with negative experiences of disclosure and is linked to victim blaming (Starzynski and Ullman, 2014).

Clearly, from this chapter you can see that blame is the single most contributing factor to negative experiences of disclosure. Ullman and Townsend (2007) found that rape myths resulting in blame attributed to the survivors often caused barriers in their interactions with a range of HCPs. This finding has been consistent in studies on disclosure to all formal support providers (Ahrens, Cabral and Abeling, 2009; Ahrens, Stansell and Jennings, 2010; Dunleavy and Slowik, 2012; Starzynski and Ullman, 2014; McQueen et al., 2021). Other negative experiences reported by survivors include HCPs' behaviour, such as minimising or dismissing responses (Ahrens, Stansell, and Jennings, 2010; McQueen, 2021) and displaying a cold and detached approach to the support (Ahrens, Cabral and Abeling, 2009). Research demonstrates that one of the key factors in positive recovery from SVA is the experience of perceived control (Peter-Hagene and Ullman, 2014). SVA can lead to decreased perceptions of personal safety, feelings of vulnerability and lower perceived control. Positive responses to disclosure that result in the survivors' experiencing perceived control after the assault is attributed to better health outcomes, lower rates of PTS and less problematic drinking reports (Orchowski, Untied and Gidycz, 2013; Ullman and Peter-Hagene, 2014). This is essential to know when considering the formal support you may give to survivors to ensure they feel empowered; thus, providing helpful short- and long-term positive recovery outcomes.

## References

Abby, A., McAuslan, P. and Ross, L. T. (1998) 'Sexual assault perpetration by college men: The role of alcohol, misperception of sexual intent, and sexual beliefs and experiences', *Journal of Social and Clinical Psychology*, 17(2), pp. 167–195.

Ahrens, C. E., Cabral, G. and Abeling, S. (2009) 'Healing or hurtful: Sexual assault survivor's interpretations of social reactions from support providers', *Psychology of Women Quarterly*, 33(1), pp. 81–94.

Ahrens, C. E., Campbell, R., Ternier-Themes, N., Wasco, S. M., and Sefl, T. (2007) 'Deciding whom to tell: Expectations and outcomes of rape survivors' first disclosures', *Psychology of Women's Quarterly*, 31, pp. 38–49.

Ahrens, E. C., Stansell, J. and Jennings, A. (2010) 'To tell or not to tell: The impact of disclosure on sexual assault Survivors' Recovery', *Violence and Victims*, 25(5), pp. 631–648.

Allen, C. T., Ridgeway, R. and Swan, S. C. (2015) 'College students' beliefs regarding help seeking for male and female sexual assault survivors: Even less support for male survivors', *Journal of Aggression Maltreatment and Trauma*, 24(1), pp. 102–115.

Allnock, D. and Miller, P. (2019). *No-One Noticed, No One Heard: A Study of Disclosures of Childhood Abuse*. London: NSPCC.

Ashmore, T., Spangaro, J. and McNamara, L. (2015) 'I was raped by Santa Claus': Responding to disclosure of sexual assault in mental health inpatient facilities', *International Journal of Mental Health Nursing*, 24(2), pp. 139–148.

Bagley, C. and King, L. (1990). *Child Sexual Abuse: The Search for Healing*. New York: Tavistock Routledge.

Berry, K. M. and Rutledge, C. M. (2016) 'Factors that influence women to disclosure sexual assault history to healthcare providers', *Journal of Obstetric, Gynaecological, and Neonatal Nursing*, 45(4), pp. 553–564.

Brownmiller, S. (1976). *Against Our Will: Men, Women, and Rape*. New York: Open Road.

Burt, M. R. (1980) 'Cultural myths and supports for rape', *Journal of Personality and Social Psychology*, 38(2), pp. 217–230.

Du Mont, J., Woldeyohannes, M., Macdonald, S., Kosa, D. and Turner, L. (2017) 'A comparison of intimate partner and other sexual assault survivors' use of different types of specialized hospital-based violence services', *BMC Women's Health*, 17(1), pp. 59–67.

Dunleavy, K. and Slowik, A. K. (2012) 'Emergence of delayed posttraumatic stress disorder symptoms related to sexual trauma: Patient-centred and trauma-cognizant management by physical therapists', *Physical Therapy*, 92(2) pp. 339–351. Available at: doi: 10.2522/ptj.20100344.

Dworkin, R. E. and Allen, N. (2018) 'Correlates of disclosure cessation after sexual assault', *Violence Against Women*, 24(1), pp. 85–100.

Filipas, H. H. and Ullman, S. E. (2001) 'Social reactions to sexual assault victims from various support sources', *Violence and Victims*, 16(6), pp. 673–692.

Fisher, B. S., Daigle, L. E., Cullen, F. T. and Turner, M. G. (2003) 'Reporting sexual victimization to the police and others: Results from a national-level study of college women', *Criminal Justice Behaviour*, 30(1), pp. 6–38.

Friedman, L. S., Samet, J. H., Roberts, M. S., Hudlin, M. and Hans, P. (1992) 'Inquiry about victimisation experiences: A survey of patient preferences and physician practices', *Archives of Internal Medicine*, 152(6), pp. 1186–1190.

Graham, R. (2006) 'Male rape and the careful construction of the male victim', *Social & Legal Studies*, 15(2), pp. 187–208.

Hakimi, D., Bryant-Davis, T., Ullman, S. and Gobin, R. L. (2018) 'Relationship between negative social reactions to sexual assault disclosure and mental health outcomes of black and white female survivors', *Psychological Trauma: Theory, Research, Practice and Psychology*, 10(3), pp. 270–275.

Heise, L. (1993). *Violence Against Women: The Missing Agenda*. In Gay, J. *The Health of Women: a global perspective*. New York: Taylor and Frances Group.

Hetu, V. (2020). "Public Attitude Towards Rape Crime and the Treatment of Its Victims in Delhi City". In Walklate, S., Fitz-Gibbon, K., Maher, J. and McCulloch, J. (Eds.), *The Emerald Handbook of Feminism, Criminology and Social Change (Emerald Studies in Criminology, Feminism and Social Change)* (pp. 137–155). Bingley: Emerald Publishing Limited.

Hollies, L. (1990). "A Daughter Survives Incest: A Retrospective Analysis". In White, E. (Ed.), *The Black Woman's Health Book: Speaking for Ourselves* (pp. 82–91). Seattle, WA: Seal Press.

Home Office (2022). *Crime outcomes in England and Wales 2021 to 2022*. Available at: https://www.gov.uk/government/statistics/crime-outcomes-in-england-and-wales-2021-to-2022/crime-outcomes-in-england-and-wales-2021-to-2022

Humphreys, C. and Thiara, R. (2003). Mental health and domestic violence: I call it symptoms of abuse', *British Journal of Social Work*, 33(2), pp. 209–226. Available at: http://dx.doi.org/10.1093/bjsw/33.2.209

Hunter, B. A., Robison, E. and Jason, L. A. (2012) 'Characteristics of sexual assault and disclosure among women in substance abuse recovery homes', *Journal of Interpersonal Violence*, 27(13), pp. 2627–2644.

Huong, T. N. (2012) 'Rape disclosure: The interplay of gender, culture and kinship in contemporary Vietnam', *Culture, Health and Sexuality*, 14(1), pp. 39–52.

Isley, P. J. (1998) 'Sexual assault of men: College age victims', *NASPA Journal*, 35(4), pp. 305–317.

Jacques-Tiura, A. J., Tkatch, R., Abbey, A. and Wegner, R. (2010) 'Disclosure of sexual assault: Characteristics and implications for posttraumatic stress symptoms among African American and Caucasian survivors', *Journal of Trauma and Dissociation*, 11(2), pp. 174–192.

Javid, A. (2017) 'Forgotten victims: Students' attitudes towards and responses to male sexual victimisation', *Journal of Sexual Aggression*, 23, pp. 338–350.

Johnson, L. M., Devereux, P. G. and Wagner, K. D. (2022) 'The group-based law enforcement mistrust scale: Psychometric properties of an adapted scale and implications for public health and harm reduction research', *Journal of Harm Reduction*, 19(40), pp. 40–56.

Khalifeh, H., Moran, P., Borchman, R., Dean, K., Hart, C., Hogg, J., Osborn, D., Johnson, S. and Howard, L. M. (2011)' Domestic and sexual violence against patients with severe mental illness', 45(4), pp 875–886

Koss, M. P. (1985) 'The hidden rape victim: Personality, attitudinal, and situational characteristics', *Psychology of Women Quarterly*, 9(2), pp. 193–212.

Koss, M. P., Dinero, T. E., Seibel, C. A. and Cox, S. L. (1988) 'Stranger and acquaintance rape: Are there differences in the victim's experience?', *Psychology of Women Quarterly*, 12(1), pp. 1–24.

Koss, M. P. (1989). Hidden rape: Sexual aggression and victimization in a national sample of students in higher education. In M. A. Pirog-Good & J. E. Stets (Eds.), *Violence in dating relationships: Emerging social issues* (pp. 145–184). New York, NY: Praeger

Krebs, C. P., Barrick, K., Lindquist, C. H., Crosby, C., Boyd, C. and Bogan, Y. (2011) 'The sexual assault of undergraduate women at historically black colleges and universities (HBCUs)', *Journal of Interpersonal Violence*, 26(18), pp. 3640–3666.

Lanthier, S., Du Mont, J. and Mason, R. (2018) 'Responding to delayed disclosure of sexual assault in health settings: A systematic review', *Journal of Trauma, Violence and Abuse*, 19(3), pp. 251–265.

Lewis, R., Marine, S. and Kenney, K. (2016) 'I get together with my friends and try to change it'. Young feminist students resist 'laddism', 'rape culture' and 'everyday sexism', *Journal of Gender Studies*, 27(1), pp. 56–72.

Lindquist, H. C., Crosby, C. M., Barrick, K., Krebs, C. P. and Settles-Reaves, B. (2016) 'Disclosure of sexual assault experiences among undergraduate women at historically black colleges and universities (HBCUs)', *Journal of American College Health*, 64(6), pp. 469–480.

Littleton, H. L., Berenson, A. B. and Breitkopf, C. R. (2007) 'An evaluation of healthcare providers' sexual violence screening practices', *American Journal of Obstetrics and Gynaecology*, 196(6), pp. 564–570.

Littleton, H. and Breitkopf, C. R. (2006) 'Coping with the experience of rape', *Psychology of Women Quarterly*, 30(1), pp. 106–116.

Logan, T., Cole, J. and Capillo, A. (2007) 'Differential characteristics of intimate partner, acquaintance, and stranger rape survivors examined by a sexual assault nurse examiner (SANE)', *Journal of Interpersonal Violence*, 22(8), pp. 1066–1076.

Lonsway, K. A. and Fitzgerald, L. F. (1994) 'Rape myths: In review', *Psychology of Women Quarterly*, 18(2), pp. 133–164.

MacKinnon, C. (1994). "Rape, Genocide and Women's Human Rights". In Stiglmayer, A. (Ed.), *Mass Rape: The War Against Women in Bosnia-Herzegovina* (pp. 183–196). Toronto: Bison Books.

McCabe, M. P. and Wauchope, M. W. (2005) 'Behavioural characteristics of men accused of rape: Evidence for different types of rapists', *Archives of Sexual Behaviour*, 34, pp. 241–253.

McLindon, E. and Harms, L. (2011) 'Listening to mental health workers' experiences: Factors influencing their work with women who disclose sexual assault', International *Journal of Mental Health Nursing*, 20, pp. 2–11.

McQueen, K., Murphy-Oikonen, J., Miller, A. and Chambers, L. (2021) 'Sexual assault: Woman's voices on the health impacts of not being believed by Police' *BMC Women's Health*, 21 https://doi.org/10.1186/s12905-021-01358-6 Available at: https://bmcwomenshealth.biomedcentral.com/articles/10.1186/s12905-021-01358-6#citeas.

Möller, A. S., Bäckström, T., Söndergaard, H. P. and Helström, L. (2012) 'Patterns of injury and reported violence depending on relationship to assailant in female Swedish sexual assault victims', *Journal of Interpersonal Violence*, 27(16), pp. 3131–3348.

Murphy, S. B., Potter, S. J., Pierce-Weeks, J., Stapleton, J. G. and Wiesen-Martin, D. (2011) 'An examination of SANE data: Clinical considerations based on victim–assailant relationship', *Journal of Forensic Nursing*, 7(3), pp. 137–144.

Orchowski, L. M., Unitied, A. S. and Gidycz, C. A. (2013) 'Social reactions to disclosure of sexual victimisation and adjustment among survivors of sexual assault', *Journal of Interpersonal Violence*, 28(10), pp. 2005–2023.

Patterson, D., Greeson, M. and Campbell, R. (2009) 'Understanding rape survivors' decisions not to seek help from formal social systems', *Health and Social Work*, 34(2), pp. 127–136.

Pennebaker, J. W. (1997) 'Writing about emotional experiences as a therapeutic process', *Psychological Science*, 8(3), pp. 162–166.

Peter, M. A. and Besley, T. (2019) 'Weinstein, sexual predation, and 'Rape Culture': Public pedagogies and the hashtag internet activism', *Education Philosophy and Theory*, 51(5), pp. 458–464.

Peter-Hagene, L. C. and Ullman, S. E. (2014) 'Social reactions to sexual assault disclosure and problem drinking: Mediating effects of perceived control and PTSD', *Journal of Interpersonal Violence*, 29(8), pp. 1418–1437.

Ranjbar, V. and Speer, S. A. (2013) 'Re-victimisation and recovery from sexual assault: Implications for health professionals', *Violence and Victims*, 28(2), pp. 274–287.

Rape Crisis England and Wales (2022) *Myths Vs Facts*. Available at: https://rapecrisis.org.uk/get-informed/about-sexual-violence/myths-vs-realities/.

Sable, M. R., Danis, F., Mauzy, D. L. and Gallagher, S. K. (2006) 'Barriers to reporting sexual assault for women and men: Perspectives of college students', *Journal of American College Health*, 55(3), pp. 157–162.

Sigurvinsdottir, R. and Ullman, S. E. (2015) 'Social reactions, self-blame, and problem drinking in adult sexual assault survivors', *Psychology of Violence*, 5(2), pp. 192–198.

Starzynski, L. L. and Ullman, S. E. (2014) 'Correlates of perceived helpfulness of mental health professionals following disclosure of sexual assault', *Violence Against Women*, 20(1), pp. 74–94.

Starzynski, L. L., Ullman, S. E., Filipas, H. H., and Townsend, S. M. (2005) 'Correlates of woman's sexual assault disclosure to informal and formal support services', *Violence and Victims*, 20(4), pp. 417–431.

Suarez, E. and Gadalla, T. M. (2010) 'Stop blaming the victim: A meta-analysis on rape myths', *Journal of Interpersonal Violence*, 25(11), pp. 2010–2035.

Tillman, S., Bryant-Davis, T., Smith, K. and Marks, A. (2010) 'Shattering silence: Exploring barriers to disclosure for African American sexual assault survivors', *Trauma Violence Abuse*, 11(2), pp. 59–70.

Turchik, J. A. and Edwards, K. M. (2012) 'Myths about male rape: A literature review', *Psychology of Men & Masculinity*, 13, pp. 211–226.

Ullman, S. E. (2011) 'Is disclosure of sexual traumas helpful? Comparing experimental laboratory verses field study Results', *Journal of Aggression, Maltreatment and Trauma*, 20(2), pp. 148–162.

Ullman, S. E. (1996) 'Social reactions, coping strategies, and self-blame attributions in adjustment to sexual assault', *Psychology of Women Quarterly*, 20(4), pp. 505–526.

Ullman, S. E. and Filipas, H. H. (2001) 'Predictors of PTSD symptom severity and social reactions in sexual assault victims', *Journal of Traumatic Stress*, 14(2), pp. 369–389.

Ullman, S. E., Foynes, M. M. and Tang, S. S. S. (2010) 'Benefits and barriers to disclosing sexual trauma: A contextual approach [Editorial]', *Journal of Trauma & Dissociation*, 11(2), pp. 127–133.

Ullman, S. E. and Najdowski, C. J. (2011) 'Prospective changes in attributions of self-blame and social reactions to women's disclosures of adult sexual assault', *Journal of Interpersonal Violence*, 26(10), pp. 1934–1962.

Ullman, S. and Peter-Hagene, L. (2014) 'Social reactions to sexual assault disclosure, coping, perceived control, and PTSD symptoms in sexual assault Victims', *Journal of Community Psychology*, 42(4), pp. 495–508.

Vandenberghe, A., Hendricks, B., Peeters, L., Roelens, K. and Keygnaert, I. (2018) 'Establishing sexual assault care centres in Belgium: Health professionals' role in the patient-centred care for victims of sexual violence', *BMC Health Services Research*, Articles number 807 https://doi.org/10.1186/s12913-018-3608-6

Walfield, S. M. (2018) '"Men cannot be raped": Correlates of male rape myth acceptance', *Journal of Interpersonal Violence*, 36(13), pp. 6319–6417.

Washington, A. P. (2001) 'Disclosure patterns of black female sexual assault survivors', *Violence Against Women*, 7(11), pp. 1254–1283.

Williston, J. C. and Lafreniere, D. K. (2013) '"Holy cow, does that ever open up a can of worms": Health care providers' experiences of inquiring about intimate partners violence', *Health Care for Woman International*, 34, pp. 814–831.

Wilson, M. (1994). *Crossing the Boundary: Black Women Survive Incest*. Seattle: Seal Press.

World Health Organisation (2013) *Responding to intimate partner violence and sexual violence against women: WHO clinical and policy guidelines*. Available at: https://apps.who.int/iris/bitstream/handle/10665/85240/9789241548595_eng.pdf.

# 4    Sexual Assault, Sexual Harassment and Stalking

## Introduction

We have discussed previously that sexual violence and abuse (SVA) is a term that is often used interchangeably, most commonly to describe many types of sexual violence. It is essential to remember that if someone has done something sexual to another person without their consent then it is, and should be, classed as sexual violence. However, the interchangeable terms used are often unhelpful for healthcare professionals that already have little knowledge around SVA or are trying to consider the best signposting support where needed. Definition and legal wise, terms are different. Whilst your service users may use one to describe the other (for example, sexual assault is the most common term to describe experiences of rape), it is important to know and understand the difference. The consequences are still devastating, for most. This chapter mentions sexual assault but really focused on the impact of sexual harassment and stalking. We feel that the first two chapter explore the sequalae of rape and sexual assault within the encompassing SVA term, therefore, don't want to be repetitive with our words.

The overarching definition of sexual (or indecent) assault that is commonly used within discourse is as follows: an act of physical, psychological and emotional violation in the form of a sexual act, inflicted on someone without their consent. It can involve forcing or manipulating someone to witness or participate in any sexual acts. They can include as follows:

- kissing.
- attempted rape.
- touching someone's breasts or genitals – including through clothing.
- touching any other part of the body for sexual pleasure or in a sexual manner – for example, stroking someone's thigh or rubbing their back.
- pressing up against another person for sexual pleasure.
- pressuring, manipulating or scaring someone into performing a sexual act on the perpetrator.
- touching someone's clothing if done for sexual pleasure or in a sexual manner – for example, lifting up someone's skirt.

(Rape Crisis, 2023)

Sexual harassment is any type of harassment involving unwanted behaviour of a sexual nature that makes a person feel distressed, intimidated or humiliated and is a sexual assault (Rape Crisis, 2022). A person does not need to have previously objected

DOI: 10.4324/9781003225461-4

to someone's behaviour for it to be considered unwanted (Citizen's Advice, 2023). Sexual harassment can include a range of actions which can include verbal, visual or physical abuse or assault. Sexual harassment may occur in a variety of settings, including at home, the workplace, in schools, nightclubs, places of worship, in organised sport, on the street, online (basically anywhere). A recent survey (All-Party Parliamentary Group [APPG] for UN Women, 2021) suggests that over 70% of women in the UK say they have experienced sexual harassment in public, this figure rises to 86% among 18–24-year-olds. Varying definitions of sexual harassment may contribute to underreporting, in the above survey only 4% formally reported the event to authorities. Sexual harassment is a worldwide problem and is primarily (although not explicitly) experienced by women from male perpetrators.

Stalking is a frequently experienced form of harassment and one of the harder crimes to define; this is partly due to stalkers using a variety of methods to harass and intimidate people, of which, many of these behaviours, taken on their own, can look innocent (Crown Prosecution Service [CPS], 2018). In the UK, it is estimated that one in five women and one in ten men will experience stalking in their adult life (Gov.UK, 2015). There are many misconceptions regarding stalking; for example, it can be perceived to have some sort of romantic element to it. Stalking is a crime and involves fixation and obsession where the attention is unwanted (CPS, 2018). Stalking is a pattern of repetitive and persistent unwanted behaviour that is intrusive and can provoke distress and fear. Stalking behaviours can include regularly sending gifts, making regular unwanted contact via telephone, text, email and/or in person (sometimes malicious), damaging a person's property and/or physical or sexual assault. Stalking can be a form of domestic abuse if the abuser is a partner or ex-partner; however, sometimes the perpetrator can also be a family member or any member of the public (CPS, 2020).

## Definitions and Terminology

As previously mentioned, defining sexual assault and stalking can be difficult due to the vast number of behaviours involved and the often-complex nature of the crime. One of the key terms in each offence is that it is unwanted behaviour, and both can cause distress, intimidation and humiliation.

## Rape

Rape is a sexual assault that involves sexual penetration. However, often defined as penetration by a penis. For example, in the UK the legal definition of rape is as follows:

1  A person (A) commits an offence if –

   a   he intentionally penetrates the vagina, anus or mouth of another person (B) with his penis,
   b   B does not consent to the penetration and
   c   A does not reasonably believe that B consents.

The legal definition of 'sexual assault' is divided into two: sexual assault and sexual assault by penetration.

**Assault by Penetration**

1   A person (A) commits an offence if –

   a   he intentionally penetrates the vagina or anus of another person (B) with a part of
       his body or anything else,
   b   the penetration is sexual,
   c   B does not consent to the penetration and
   d   A does not reasonably believe that B consents.

**Sexual Assault**

1   A person (A) commits an offence if –

   a   he intentionally touches another person (B),
   b   the touching is sexual,
   c   B does not consent to the touching and
   d   A does not reasonably believe that B consents.

All three definitions carry section 2 relating to consent:

2   Whether a belief is reasonable is to be determined having regard to all the circum-
    stances, including any steps A has taken to ascertain whether B consents.

(legislation.gov.uk, 2023)

**Sexual Harassment**

Over the years, various definitions of sexual harassment have disagreed on: whether a
power differential is necessary; whether a location needs to be specified; the importance
placed on whether the survivor perceives the behaviour as problematic; whether only
women can be sexually harassed; whether an act can be defined as harassing in and of
itself or whether further negative consequences are necessary for the act to be a legiti-
mate case of sexual harassment; and lastly whether sexist (e.g., 'gender harassment' as
opposed to sexual) behaviour is a type of sexual harassment O'Donohue, Downs and
Yeater, 1998).
   Sexual harassment can include but is not limited to:

- sexually degrading comments or gestures
- your body being stared or leered at
- being subjected to sexual jokes or propositions
- emails or text messages with sexual content
- physical behaviour, including unwelcome sexual advances, aggressive/unwanted touching and rape
- someone displaying sexually explicit pictures in your space or a shared space, like at
  work
- taking and circulating sexual photos
- forced viewing of pornography
- offers of rewards in return for sexual favours
- stalking

(Rape Crisis, 2022 and APPG for UN Women, 2021)

In effect, sexual harassment is *unwelcome sexual conduct* (APPG for UN Women, 2021). Due to sexual harassment occurring in a variety of environments, often there are definitions and terminology based on the place of the crime, for example, online sexual harassment, workplace sexual harassment, domestic abuse. These will be discussed further later in this chapter.

## Stalking

Although stalking can sometimes be seen as a type of sexual harassment, it is important to look at this definition separately as it involves unique behaviours and legislation. Early definitions of stalking were concerned mainly with the behaviour of the perpetrator, however since the mid-1990s literature extended this to include the reaction of and impact on the survivor (Meloy and Gothard, 1995; Mullen et al., 1999). It is commonly accepted that stalking is a behaviour of persistence usually occurring on at least two separate occasions (Purcell, Pathé and Mullen, 2004; Gowland, 2013). Taylor-Dunn, Bowen and Gilchrist (2021) argue that it is the impact on the survivor, which makes stalking difficult to define as the perpetrator's behaviour may appear harmless. However, these seemingly harmless behaviours can have a devastating impact on the survivor when taken in context of the wider pattern of behaviours (Taylor-Dunn, Bowen and Gilchrist, 2021).

In the majority of stalking and harassment cases, there will be some connection between the survivor and the suspect, even if the survivor is unaware of who the suspect is (for example, where they have only briefly met in passing). Behaviour by a perpetrator could include as follows: following or watching/spying on a person; contacting, or attempting to contact a person by any means, for example, attending at the home or the workplace of the person, telephone calls, text messages, emails or use of other mechanisms such as the internet and social networking sites; monitoring the persons use of phone/internet (for example, emails); sending letters or unwanted 'gifts' to the person or arranging for others to deliver items to the person; damaging the person's property; boasting that they are aware of the location or address of other family members or children; burglary or robbery of the person's possessions; becoming further and further embedded within a person's life, for example, by making contact with their friends and family; threats of physical harm to the person (including sexual violence and threats to kill); physical and/or sexual assault of the person and even murder (Sheridan and Davies, 2001; Women's Aid, 2021).

Mullen and Pathé (2002) have previously identified six main types of survivors; they are dependent on their previous relationship to the stalker: Table 4.1 highlights the different types of survivors.

*Table 4.1* Stalking: Types of Survivors

| | Survivor Type | Description |
|---|---|---|
| 1 | Prior intimates | Survivors who have been in a previous intimate relationship with their stalker |
| 2 | Casual acquaintances and friends | Friends or people you have met socially |
| 3 | Professional contacts | Survivors who have been stalked by patients, clients or students who they have had a professional relationship with |
| 4 | Workplace contacts | Either an employer, employee or a customer |
| 5 | Strangers | People who are unknown to them |
| 6 | Famous/celebrities | People who are widely known, who receives acclaim and attention |

*Table 4.2* Stalking: Types of Perpetrators

|   | Perpetrator Type | Description |
|---|---|---|
| 1 | Rejected stalkers | are motivated in order to reverse, correct or avenge a rejection (e.g., divorce, separation, termination) |
| 2 | Resentful stalkers | are usually motivated by the desire to frighten and distress the survivor due to a sense of grievance |
| 3 | Intimacy seekers | aim to establish an intimate, loving relationship with their survivor. Such stalkers often believe they were 'meant' to be together |
| 4 | Incompetent suitors | often have a fixation on a person and sometimes a sense of entitlement to an intimate relationship with someone that has attracted their interest; however, this type of stalker often has poor social or courting skills, and their survivors are most often already in a dating relationship with someone else |
| 5 | Predatory stalkers | are motivated to spy on the survivor in order to prepare and plan an attack – often a sexual crime |

Mullen and Pathé (2002) suggest that the most common type of survivor is a prior intimate, usually a woman who has previously shared an intimate relationship with her (usually) male stalker. These survivors are more likely to be exposed to violence being enacted by their stalker especially if the stalker had a criminal past.

As for the perpetrators, there can be different motivating factors which prompt their behaviour. These can include but are not limited to: revenge; retribution; loneliness; resentment; a desire for reconciliation; response to a perceived insult or humiliation; or a desire for control. They may also demonstrate delusional belief that an individual is in love with them (termed 'erotomania'), and that sooner or later they will reciprocate (CPS, 2018). Mullen, Pathé, Purcell and Stuart (1999) also identified types of stalkers which are now generally accepted terms. Table 4.2 illustrates the different types of stalkers.

What is agreed is that stalking is persistent and unwanted attention by an individual or group that makes a person feel pestered and harassed. It may cause them to feel alarmed or distressed or to fear that violence might be used against them (Pathé and Mullen, 1997; Spitzberg and Cupach, 2007).

## Historical Context in the UK

### Sexual Assault

The historical context of SVA is explored briefly in Chapter 2. It is important to recognise that what is known about the history of sexual assault (SVA) is only known from to period it became a crime. As this point there were records of its reporting. However, and as previously emphasised, reporting was and remains a very small insight into experience or awareness due to the lack of reporting/disclosure. D'Cruze writes very thoroughly on the history of SVA in the Handbook of Sexual Violence (Brown and Walklate, 2012). We would recommend this chapter if you would like an in-depth analysis of the history of SVA throughout the 15th century to present times. It does not impact the way you support survivors; however, it gives great insight into how a patriarchal society and culture of sexually has influenced and shaped the way we see SVA in modern society; this, therefore, directly effects how we respond to disclosures.

It would not surprise you to know that whilst supportive mechanism has improved, the invisibly of SVA is a thread that continues to follow us into the 21st century. For example, when considering the statistics and the impact of SVA on health, think about how much focus was given to this topic in your education/training for your profession compared to that of other health conditions such as stroke, coronary care, smoking and substance abuse.

## Sexual Harassment

Although sexual harassment has become more publicly discussed worldwide over the last few years, it has been recognised as a problem and has been in existence for a long time in every part of society. However, the term 'sexual harassment' has only been discussed in literature and media since the 1970s (Gardner, 1972; Kamberi and Gollopeni, 2015). Throughout the years, studies have consistently shown that a significant number of women and girls have experienced sexual harassment in their lives, and it continues to be a major problem worldwide. The numbers presented have often varied; this may be due to underreporting, and thus, historically data has underrepresented the number of women affected (APPG for UN Women, 2021).

In the UK, it was only in 1986 that the Sexual Discrimination Act (SDA) of 1975 was modified to establish sexual harassment as a form of discrimination, although interestingly the Act does not specifically mention sexual harassment as a term, the Court of Session declared that sexual harassment may be a form of direct sex discrimination (The Sex Discrimination Act [SDA], 1986; Lockwood, Rosenthal and Budjanovcanin, 2006). It was not until 2005 that the Employment Equality Sex Discriminations Regulations stated that 'sexual harassment occurs where there is unwanted conduct of a sexual nature that violates a person's dignity, or creates an intimidating, hostile, degrading, humiliating or offensive environment for them. If an employer treats someone less favourably because they have rejected, or submitted to, form of harassment described above, this is also harassment'. Today, sexual harassment at work is covered by the Equality Act (2010). The law now defines sexual harassment more broadly as a behaviour that makes a person feel intimidated or offended, related to their sex. Although this Act is in place, many organisations and charities are pushing the government to put policies in place due to the prevalence of sexual harassment in the workplace.

## Stalking

'Prowler' or 'poacher' has been used as terms since at least the 16th century to describe 'someone who secretly follows people or hides near their houses, especially at night, in order to steal something, frighten them, or perhaps harm them' (Collins Dictionary, 2005). The term 'stalker' has only been used more recently in the 20th century to describe people who harass and pester others; initially the term was related to the harassment of celebrities by strangers (Pathé, Mullen and Purcell, 2001). With time, the meaning and understanding of stalking changed to include individuals being harassed by their former partners (Mullen and Pathé, 2002). It was not until 2012 that the UK government created a law specifically aimed at stalking. The Protection of Harassment Act of 1997 was updated to include the offence of stalking in England and Wales. Although stalking is considered illegal in most parts of the world, some of the actions that contribute to stalking may be legal, such as gathering information, calling or texting someone, sending gifts, emailing, or direct messaging over social media, often making it difficult for the recipient to report and determine the severity of the crime (APPG for UN Women, 2021).

## Current Context

Sexual harassment has been thrust to the fore over the last five years; it has been highlighted in the media as a result of the 2017 #Metoo and #TimesUp campaigns in which many top-profile celebrities came forward and exposed sexual harassment in the workplace, thus giving many more people a platform to start discussing and reporting sexual harassment cases. More recently in the UK, a very high-profile rape and murder case involving a woman named Sarah Everard created a swift rise in awareness and discussion around the deep-rooted problems with authorities such as the police force and sexual harassment. However, a positive arising from such high-profile cases often gives others the confidence to speak up and come forward about their own experience and help the general public understand the seriousness of these crimes.

As mentioned previously, a recent survey (APPG for UN Women, 2021) of 1,089 women in the UK reported that 71% of women of all ages had experienced some form of sexual harassment in a public space (86% among 18–24-year-olds). 'Public space' was defined as any of the following: public transport (buses, trains, etc.), hospitality venues (pubs, clubs, bars, etc.), public events (concerts, sports games, festivals, etc.), streets, parks, commons and other public recreational spaces and online spaces (social media). The survey highlighted that the most common forms of sexual harassment of those listed are being cat-called or wolf-whistled (51%), being stared at (44%), and unwelcome touching, body rubbing or groping (37%). Moreover, the list of behaviours was not exhaustive nor was there the option of 'other', so of the 20% who answered 'none of these' suggests there may be some who had experienced some other form of sexual harassment in a public space. Prior to the study in 2021, a YouGov (YouGov, 2017) survey highlighted a lesser number (7% less) of women of all ages across the UK are experiencing sexual harassment in a public place (64%). This could be due to a number of reasons already mentioned – it would appear that sexual harassment may have increased during the COVID-19 pandemic but also because of the high-profile campaigns of 2017, #MeToo and #TimesUp public awareness and understanding of what sexual harassment is, has increased, meaning women may feel more comfortable stating their experience as sexual harassment than before. A study by Plan International UK and Our Streets Now (2020) revealed that 19% of girls aged 14–21 in the UK had experienced public sexual harassment since the start of the lockdown, 28% of women/girls reported feeling less safe going out in public now than they did before the lockdown (Plan International UK, 2020).

Not only is sexual harassment recognised in public spaces, but it is also equally prolific in places of work and study. A study carried out by the Trades Union Congress (2016) entitled 'Still just a bit of banter?' revealed that over half of women in the UK have experienced sexual harassment while at work. They surveyed over 1,500 women and discovered that 52% have been survivors of unwanted sexual behaviours at work, for women aged 16–24 this percentage rose to 63%, with almost 20% of women reporting that the person harassing them was their manager or someone in a position of authority. Workplace sexual harassment although being tackled by many organisations is still widespread across all sectors and is a worldwide problem. When considering workplace harassment, we must remember that this is not just an issue for women who work in offices (which is often portrayed in TV shows or movies), but rather we must expand our thinking to the wider workforce; there are many studies showing the appalling numbers of women experiencing sexual harassment in the armed forces, police force, commercial travel industry, hospitality and tourism, healthcare, sciences and many more (Godier and Fossey, 2018; Ross et al., 2019; Sweeting, Arabaci-Hills and Cole, 2021).

The APPG for UN Women (2021) survey did not include places of work or study which we know are two of the most common places for sexual harassment. A noteworthy point is that this study took place during the COVID-19 pandemic; therefore, the lack of workplace inclusion is not surprising as these areas where impacted the most during the pandemic. However, a recent study (Rights of women, 2021) demonstrated that during the pandemic, workplace sexual harassment continued to be an issue for women working from home, and for some even worsened. They found that 45% of women experiencing sexual harassment reported experiencing the harassment remotely, for example, sexual messages (email, texts, social media); cyber harassment (via Zoom, Teams, Slack etc.) and sexual calls. These incidents likely increased as people spent more time online during lockdowns throughout the pandemic.

*Online Sexual Harassment*

The last 20 years have seen an exponential increase in the use of technology and with that comes the increased accessibility to digital platforms, digital services and digital information. The UK holds one of the highest internet penetration rates across the world, with approximately 63 million monthly users in 2021 which is expected to rise to over 65 million monthly users by 2026 (Statista, 2023). In a progressively digital world, the use of online platforms and social media increases, and so too does technology-facilitated sexual violence (TFSV), a broad term coined by Henry and Powell (2015) to capture the array of harms facilitated through technology (Setty, Ringrose and Regehr, 2023). Under the term TFSV, image-based sexual abuse (McGlynn and Rackley, 2017) or 'revenge porn' as it is widely referred to, any non-consensual digital practices (Henry and Powell, 2018) and online sexual harassment are included.

Online sexual harassment is defined as any unwanted sexual behaviour on any digital platform (Project deSHAME, 2019). It can take place between anyone online and includes an array of behaviours that use digital content (videos, messages, post, images, webpages) placed on a range of online platforms both private and public. A noteworthy point is that very often, multiple platforms are used simultaneously to share the information, thus heightening the impact of sexual harassment online. Equally, online sexual harassment does not always happen in isolation and very often overlaps between the online and offline worlds (Project deSHAME, 2019). The UN Women UK survey (APPG for UN Women, 2021) found that 17% of women in the UK experienced online comments or jokes that made them feel unsafe or uncomfortable and 14% experienced sharing of suggestive, indecent, or unsolicited content online or in person. In a study conducted by Cybersmile (2017), 30% of women stated they had seen bullying or harassment online, with Facebook and Twitter being two of the main platforms where the female respondents saw the most bullying and harassment (Cybersmile, 2017). An Amnesty International survey in 2017 found that 21% of women had experienced online abuse, of which 27% received threats of physical or sexual violence, 47% received sexist or misogynistic comments and 69% received generally abusive language or comments. 'Cyber flashing' is another common form of sexual harassment online. A YouGov survey in 2018 found that 19% of all women and 40% of women aged 18–34 have received an unsolicited sexual photo from someone who is not a romantic partner (YouGov, 2018). In addition, the UK's Revenge Porn Helpline reported a rise in calls by 87% about explicit imagery being shared without consent between April and August 2020 versus the previous year (SWGFL Safe, Secure, Online, 2021).

*Stalking*

As mentioned earlier, in the UK, it is estimated that one in five women and one in ten men will experience stalking in their adult life (Gov.UK, 2015), although this is believed to be grossly underestimated due to underreporting. As mentioned previously reporting of harassment and stalking is minimal; it has been estimated previously that survivors of stalking do not tend to report to the police until the 100th incident (Network for Surviving Stalking, 2009). This means that a large proportion of survivors will never expose their experience. The majority of survivors are female, while the majority of perpetrators are male (NAPO, 2011). Although this is a crime mainly by men against women, it is important to note that women often target other women, and males report being stalked by both females and males alike (Pathé and Mullen, Purcell, 2001).

It is important to note that cultural norms can affect the way stalking is perceived, making it difficult to define and understand what is considered culturally acceptable. Previous literature suggests that many men and women admit engaging in various stalking-like behaviours following a romantic break-up (Langhinrichsen-Rohling, 2012); however, this behaviour usually stops over time. Langhinrichsen-Rohling (2012) suggests that it can be normal within heterosexual dating relationships for engagement in low levels of unwanted pursuit behaviours to be displayed for a relatively short amount of time, particularly in the context of a relationship break-up. This can make it difficult to decern unwanted 'normative' behaviour in contrast to behaviour that is unwanted and dangerous. Surveillance is becoming increasingly easier with the introduction of new technologies that connect users' devices with everyday objects (e.g., findmyfriends applications, home security systems, internet-connected home assistants like Amazon echo). Given the ubiquity of technology, some degree of social surveillance (such as monitoring an intimate partner's social media accounts) may be considered an acceptable part of relationships (Marwick, 2012). This can make identifying and reporting of stalking difficult, especially for those who have recently experienced a relationship break-up. Furthermore, studies across the globe have demonstrated significant barriers in the reporting of stalking to the police and show that police can be unhelpful, with survivors being subject to a victim-blaming response (Taylor-Dunn, Bowen and Gilchrist, 2021).

Stalking can take place in person, on the phone or over the internet, the latter is known as 'cyberstalking' and can include the use of emails, social networking sites, chat rooms and other forums facilitated by technology (Kaur et al., 2021). Cyberstalking has become a huge concern in recent decades as use of the internet has become readily available, quicker and more private. Defined by an individual's digital skills, cyberstalking has also made some people more exposed through the use of social media, which if used naively makes available peoples 'online profiles', in which personal information is shared openly. The internet opens up greater opportunities for gathering information which can be used for a range of purposes relating to stalking and harassment, for example: to find personal information about someone, as a means of surveillance, to communicate with the person, damaging someone's reputation and sending unwanted sexual images (CPS, 2018). Excessive use of technology-enabled communication platforms has led to an increased awareness of rising incidents of cyberstalking but again scholars have found this crime difficult to define due to its various forms (Kaur et al., 2021).

During the COVID-19 pandemic, government policies, including lockdowns and social distancing, escalated the frequency and associated risks of stalking. Perpetrators were more likely to be aware of survivors' locations because of their restricted movements. Furthermore, many healthcare facilities, charities and public sector organisations had restricted services, further compounding the situation. The stalking advocacy service Veritas Justice reported a 26% increase in referrals since the first lockdown period in March 2020 compared to their previous three-month average (Sussex Police and Crime Commissioner, 2021). Other UK-based advocacy agencies including Paladin and the Suzy Lamplugh Trust reported similar findings, with a surge in cyberstalking during the first four weeks of lockdown.

It is clear from the literature that many women do not formally report their experiences of sexual harassment whether it be in person or online to authorities. The UN women survey (APPG for UN Women, 2021) found that over 95% of all women did not formally report their experiences. The two main reasons women of all ages cited for not reporting incidents are as follows: 'I didn't think the incident was serious enough to report' (55%) and 'I didn't think reporting it would help' (45%). Furthermore, if women do report the incident, figures show that only few (16%) cases recorded by the police will actually result in a charge prosecution. Figures for stalking are even worse, only 1% of cases of stalking recorded by the police result in a charge and prosecution by the Crown Prosecution Service (CPS) (Paladin National Stalking Advocacy Service, 2015).

## Impact of Sexual Harassment and Stalking

### The Survivor

The impact that these particular crimes can have on a person varies considerably especially when you take into account the vast array of behaviours and situations involved. Survivors can suffer, physical, psychological and social and financial effects (Messing et al., 2020). Disruptions in daily life necessary to escape these threatening and intimidating behaviours can have a negative impact on the survivor's well-being. During the episodes of such behaviours, they may feel a whole raft of emotions such as feeling scared, threatened, humiliated, degraded, isolated, guilty and judged.

A review by Spitzberg and Cupach (2007) identified several effects that stalking can have on a person, including but not limited to emotional/psychological impact such as post-traumatic stress (PTS), anger, anxiety, depression, fear, jealousy and paranoia. Physical health effects can take the form of addictions, appetite or sleep disturbance, and changes in lifestyle patterns. Financial costs include accessing counselling, time taken off work and moving to get away from the perpetrator. There is also the social impact – where the behaviours can affect close contacts of the survivor – friends may need to adapt schedules to accommodate the survivor, co-workers may have to compensate for missed work, and, in some cases, those who help survivors may also become targets of the stalker themselves. Research demonstrates strong associations between stalking victimisation and harmful effects along multiple dimensions of these symptoms (Spitzberg and

Cupach, 2007; Messing et al., 2020). It must be highlighted that sometimes presuming causation is not always the correct way to approach certain effects – some of these difficulties may have preceded the stalking which may have promoted relationship dissolution; stalking can occasionally emerge out of a dysfunctional relational system (Spitzberg and Cupach, 2007).

### The Family of Survivors

As well as the survivor themselves, stalking can also have a direct impact on the survivor's family and close friends. It is common for friends and family to be abused by a stalker attempting to gain access to their primary target, causing social isolation (Eterovic-Soric et al., 2017). Family members can develop depression or stress disorders as they worry about the person (Riger, Raja and Camacho, 2002). The perpetrators' manipulative behaviour often isolates the person being abused further; for example, some studies have shown that the perpetrator can make life difficult for the survivor and their supporters (family and friends) and also in the survivor's place of work – sometimes leading to the survivor's unemployment further isolation and economic difficulty (Messing et al., 2020).

### The Wider Society

The effects of sexual harassment and stalking are not restricted to the individual and their family as the individual lives in a larger social system. Sexual harassment and stalking victimisation often carry unseen costs (Spitzberg and Cupach, 2007); for example, the survivors use of policing and the judicial system (for example to address a proximity violation of a restraining order) draws upon police resources; healthcare visits due to physical and psychological needs can draw upon NHS resources; and days missed at work can impact employment productivity.

## Current Legal Position and Policies Response

The number of sexual offences recorded by the police within the UK has been at an all-time high; however, the percentage of those being reported that result in conviction has been falling sharply for six year, resulting in an all-time low. It is important to acknowledge that these figures are made public and often result in headlining news, therefore, not only destroying survivors faith in the justice system but also acting as a deterrent for those considering disclosing; barriers you may see in practice.

Sexual harassment and stalking are illegal. Although legislation was first introduced in California, USA, in 1990, prompted by the case of an actress stalked and then murdered by an obsessed fan (Gilligan, 1992; Tjaden, 2009), it was not until 2012 that the UK government updated The Protection of Harassment Act of 1997 and created a law specifically aimed at stalking. The Protection from Harassment Act (1997) outlines harassment as 'causing alarm or distress' (section 2), and 'putting people in fear of violence' (section 4). For it to be considered 'harassment' the behaviour must happen on more than one occasion by the same person or group; however, it is worth noting that the behaviours can vary on each occasion. The Protection of Freedoms Act (2012) included two new offences; section 2A: stalking, defined as harassment which involves a course of conduct that amounts to stalking; and section 4A: stalking which can be committed two ways: stalking involving fear of violence or stalking involving serious alarm or distress. According to the CPS, stalking cases remain, 'difficult to prosecute' (CPS, 2018). Consistently, current stalking laws rely on the survivors' sense of fear and the survivor reporting to police a belief that the stalker will cause physical harm (Storey and Hart, 2011; Cheyne and Guggisberg, 2018). Ultimately, it then resides with the courts to decide if something is deemed harassment or stalking under the Act. The courts base the decision on whether a reasonable person would interpret the magnitude of behaviours as harassment.

Survivors who experience harassment hold the right to apply for an injunction. An injunction can forbid a perpetrator from doing certain things such as contacting the person directly or indirectly, going to their home address, place of work or children's school. Survivors may also seek a restraining order, the breach of which may lead to a criminal offence. It is worth noting. However, that no power of arrest can be attached to this civil order. So, in order to enforce it through the civil courts, the survivor is required to return to court and apply for a warrant of arrest. If the survivor is associated to the perpetrator, they may have the option to apply to the Family Court for a domestic violence injunction, namely a non-molestation order. In cases where sexual harassment takes place within the workplace, the legal position may vary as it is an issue of illegal employment discrimination. Workplace sexual harassment may be considered illegal when it creates a hostile or offensive work environment or when it results in an adverse employment decision, such as the survivor's demotion, firing or quitting. For any survivor of stalking or harassment, it is important that they know their options and are encouraged to seek appropriate legal guidance and advice.

## Supporting Survivors

If someone presents in the healthcare system and discloses experiencing sexual harassment or stalking, it is important that this is taken seriously and in line with the correct system policies and protocols. This is discussed in Chapter 10 (supporting survivors). Specific organisations available to signpost for help and support are as follows:

Gov.uk – https://www.gov.uk/report-stalker
National stalking helpline – https://www.suzylamplugh.org/Pages/Category/national-stalking-helpline
Paladin service – https://www.paladinservice.co.uk/
Protection against stalking – https://www.protectionagainststalking.org/
Women's aid – https://www.womensaid.org.uk/information-support/what-is-domestic-abuse/stalking/
Support line – https://www.supportline.org.uk/problems/stalking-and-harassment/
Police.UK – https://www.police.uk/advice/advice-and-information/sh/stalking-harassment/support-victims-harassment/
Victim support – https://www.victimsupport.org.uk/crime-info/types-crime/stalking-and-harassment/
My support space – https://www.mysupportspace.org.uk/moj
Revenge porn helpline – https://revengepornhelpline.org.uk/
Enough campaign – https://enough.campaign.gov.uk/what-is-abuse

**Case Study 1**

Fiona is a 32-year-old female and mother of three young children (3, 4 and 8). Fiona presented at the GP surgery with symptoms of depression and anxiety. It was also clear that she had cut marks on her arms which she was not trying to cover up. She mentioned at the consultation that her husband and she were going through a divorce and that she has found it very difficult – especially as she desires her children to have contact with their father to maintain the relationship between them. She mentions that she is becoming increasingly frightened by his erratic behaviour and the lies that he has told her when he comes to pick up the children. She says that he has often been seen around the house when it is not his 'turn' to have the children and this has worried her. She thinks he may be stalking her and have access to her email and social media accounts. He seems to know details of what she has been doing and where she has been when he comes to collect the children. He has never abused the children that she is aware of but recently the eldest has mentioned that he has been swearing a lot and being nasty about Fiona in front of the children. She mentioned that he has been lying to the wider family about why their relationship broke down and she feels he is trying to turn them against her.

**How would you support Fiona, what advice would you give?**

....................................................................................................................

....................................................................................................................

....................................................................................................................

....................................................................................................................

....................................................................................................................

....................................................................................................................

....................................................................................................................

....................................................................................................................

....................................................................................................................

....................................................................................................................

....................................................................................................................

....................................................................................................................

**Case Study 2**

A university student (Anya) studying physics attends the sexual health clinic for a routine check-up. She seems worried. During the assessment, Anya discloses that she had consensual penetrative sex with one of her university tutors. Following this Anya's tutor has requested a number of individual tutorial/meetings with her outside of university hours and she is worried about how to say no to the tutor as she feels if she refuses it will have a negative impact on her studies.

**How would you support Anya, what advice would you give?**

..................................................................................................................

..................................................................................................................

..................................................................................................................

..................................................................................................................

..................................................................................................................

..................................................................................................................

..................................................................................................................

..................................................................................................................

..................................................................................................................

..................................................................................................................

..................................................................................................................

..................................................................................................................

..................................................................................................................

..................................................................................................................

..................................................................................................................

..................................................................................................................

..................................................................................................................

# References

All-Party Parliamentary Group (APPG) for UN Women (2021) Prevalence and Reporting of Sexual Harassment in UK Public Spaces. https://www.unwomenuk.org/site/wp-content/uploads/2021/03/APPG-UN-Women-Sexual-Harassment-Report_Updated.pdf

Cheyne, N. and Guggisberg, M. (2018) "Stalking: An Age Old Problem with New Expressions in the Digital Age". In Guggisberg, M. and Henricksen, J. (Eds.), *Violence Against Women in the 21st Century: Challenges and Future Directions* (pp. 161–190). Hauppauge, NY: Nova Science Publishers.

Citizen's Advice (2023) Check What You Can Do about Harassment. Available at: https://www.citizensadvice.org.uk/law-and-courts/discrimination/what-are-the-different-types-of-discrimination/sexual-harassment/

Collins Dictionary (2005) Definition of 'Prowler'. Penguin Random House LLC. Available at: https://www.collinsdictionary.com/dictionary/english/prowler

Crown Prosecution Service (CPS) (2018) Stalking and Harassment. Available at: https://www.cps.gov.uk/legal-guidance/stalking-and-harassment

Crown Prosecution Service (CPS) (2020) Stalking Analysis Reveals Domestic Abuse Link. Available at: https://www.cps.gov.uk/cps/news/stalking-analysis-reveals-domestic-abuse-link

Cybersmile (2017) Stop Cyberbullying Day Survey 2017. Available at: https://www.cybersmile.org/wp-content/uploads/Stop-Cyberbullying-Day-Survey2017.pdf

Equality Act 2010: Guidance (2010) *Equality Act 2010*. Available at: https://www.gov.uk/guidance/equality-act-2010-guidance

Eterovic-Soric, B., Choo, K. K. R., Ashman, H. and Mubarak, S. (2017) 'Stalking the stalkers–detecting and deterring stalking behaviours using technology: A review', *Computers & Security*, 70, pp. 278–289.

Gardner, H. (1972) '…and every prisoner an unprintable word', *The Globe and Mail*, 18 March 1972, p. 35. Source: ProQuest Historical Newspapers digital archive.

Gilligan, M. J. (1992) 'Stalking the stalker: Developing new laws to thwart those who terrorize others', *Georgia Law Review*, 27, p. 285.

Godier, L. R. and Fossey, M. (2018) 'Addressing the knowledge gap: Sexual violence and harassment in the UK armed forces', *BMJ Military Health*, 164(5), pp. 362–364.

Gov.UK (2015) New Measures to Protect Victims of Stalking, Domestic Abuse and Violence. Available at: https://www.gov.uk/government/news/new-measures-to-protect-victims-of-stalking-domestic-abuse-and-violence

Gov.UK (2019) Consultation On Sexual Harassment in the Workplace. Available at: https://www.gov.uk/government/consultations/consultation-on-sexual-harassment-in-the-workplace

Gowland, J. (2013) 'Protection from Harassment Act 1997: The 'New' stalking offences', *The Journal of Criminal Law*. 77(5), pp. 387–398. https://doi.org/10.1350/jcla.2013.77.5.865

Henry, N. and Powell, A. (2015) 'Technology-facilitated sexual violence and harassment against women', *Australia and New Zealand Journal of Criminology*, 448(1), pp. 104–118.

Henry, N. and Powell, A. (2018) 'Technology-facilitated sexual violence: A literature review of empirical research', *Trauma, Violence and Abuse*, 19(2), pp. 195–208.

Kamberi, F. and Gollopeni, B. (2015) 'The phenomenon of sexual harassment at the workplace in Republic of Kosovo', *International Review of Social Sciences*, 3(12), pp. 580–592.

Kaur, P., Dhir, A., Tandon, A., Alzeiby, E. A. and Abohassan, A. A. (2021) 'A systematic literature review on cyberstalking. An analysis of past achievements and future promises', *Technological Forecasting and Social Change*, 163, p. 120426.

Langhinrichsen-Rohling, J. (2012) 'Gender and stalking: Current intersections and future directions', *Sex Roles*, 66(5), pp. 418–426.

Lockwood, G., Rosenthal, P. and Budjanovcanin, A. (2006) 'Sexual harassment and the law: The British experience', *Managerial Law*, 48(5), pp. 455–466.

Marwick, A. (2012) 'The public domain: Surveillance in everyday life', *Surveillance & Society*, 9(4), pp. 378–393.

McGlynn, C. and Rackley, E. (2017) 'Image-based sexual abuse', *Oxford Journal of Legal Studies*, 37(3), pp. 534–561.

Meloy, J. and Gothard, S. (1995) 'Demographic and clinical comparison of obsessional followers and offenders with mental disorders', *The American Journal of Psychiatry*, 152. pp. 258–263. https://doi.org/10.1176/ajp.152.2.258

Messing, J., Bagwell-Gray, M., Brown, M. L., Kappas, A. and Durfee, A. (2020) 'Intersections of stalking and technology-based abuse: Emerging definitions, conceptualization, and measurement', *Journal of Family Violence*, 35(7), pp. 693–704.

Mullen, P. E. and Pathé, M. (2002) 'Stalking', *Crime and Justice*, 29, pp. 273–318.

Mullen, P. E., Pathé, M., Purcell, R. and Stuart, G. W. (1999) Study of stalkers. *American Journal of Psychiatry*, 156(8), pp. 1244–1249. https://doi.org/10.1176/ajp.156.8.1244

NAPO (2011) Stalking and Harassment – A Study of Perpetrators. Available at: https://www.napo.org.uk/sites/default/files/BRF22-11%20Stalking%20and%20Harassment%20-%20a%20study%20of%20perpetrators.pdf

Network for Surviving Stalking (2009) Stalking Survey Findings Report. London, England. Available at: https://www.officeforstudents.org.uk/advice-and-guidance/student-information-and-data/national-student-survey-nss/

O'Donohue, W., Downs, K. and Yeater, E. A. (1998) 'Sexual harassment: A review of the literature', *Aggression and Violent Behavior*, 3(2), pp. 111–128.

Paladin National Stalking Advocacy Service (2015) Paladin Briefing: Key Headlines from the Report 'Stalking Law: Two Years on November 2012-2014'. Available at: https://studylib.net/doc/6654039/key-headlines-from-the-stalking-law--two-years-on

Pathé, M. and Mullen, P. E. (1997) 'The impact of stalkers on their victims', *The British Journal of Psychiatry*, 170(1), pp. 12–17.

Plan International UK (2020) The State of Girls' Rights in the UK – Early Insights into the Impact of the Coronavirus Pandemic on Girls. Available at: https://plan-uk.org/file/plan-uk-state-of-girls-rights-coronavirus-reportpdf

Project deSHAME (2019) Online Sexual Harassment. Understand, Prevent and Respond. Available at: https://hwb.gov.wales/api/storage/b51d7fc2-49e2-4b01-ade4-12b05b64daec/Handbook_Senior_Management_WALES_Print%20-%20English.pdf

Protections Against Freedoms Act (2012) Protection Against Freedom Act. Available at: https://www.legislation.gov.uk/ukpga/2012/9/contents/enacted

Purcell, R., Pathé, M. and Mullen, P. E. (2001) 'A study of women who stalk', *American Journal of Psychiatry*, 158(12), pp. 2056–2060.

Rape Crisis. (2022) What Is Sexual Harassment? Available at: https://rapecrisis.org.uk/get-informed/types-of-sexual-violence/what-is-sexual-harassment/

Rape Crisis (2023) *What is Sexual Assault.* Available at: https://rapecrisis.org.uk/get-informed/types-of-sexual-violence/what-is-sexual-assault/

Riger, S., Raja, S. and Camacho, J. (2002) 'The radiating impact of intimate partner violence', *Journal of Interpersonal Violence*, 17(2), pp. 184–205.

Rights of Women (2021) Rights of Women – Helping Women through the Law. Available at: https://rightsofwomen.org.uk/news/rights-of-women-survey-reveals-online-sexual-harassment-has-increased-as-women-continue-to-suffer-sexual-harassment-whilst-working-through-the-covid-19-pandemic/

Ross, S., Naumann, P., Hinds-Jackson, D. V. and Stokes, L. (2019) Sexual Harassment in Nursing: Ethical Considerations and Recommendations. *OIJN Online Journal. Issues in Nursing*, 24(1), pp. 1–13.

Setty, E., Ringrose, J. and Regehr, K. (2023) "Chapter 4: Digital Sexual Violence and the Gendered Constraints of Consent in Youth Image Sharing". In Horvath, M. A. H. and Brown, J. M. (Eds.), *Rape: Challenging Contemporary Thinking – 10 Years On*. Oxon: Taylor Francis Group.

Sheridan, L. and Davies, G. M. (2001) 'Stalking: The elusive crime', *Legal and Criminological Psychology*, 6(2), pp. 133–147.

Spitzberg, B. H. and Cupach, W. R. (2007) 'The state of the art of stalking: Taking stock of the emerging literature', *Aggression and Violent Behavior*, 12(1), pp. 64–86.

Statista (2023) Internet Usage in the United Kingdom (UK) – Statistics and Facts. Available at: https://www.statista.com/topics/3246/internet-usage-in-the-uk/#topicOverview

Storey, J. E. and Hart, S. D. (2011) 'How Do Police Respond to Stalking? An Examination of the Risk Management Strategies and Tactics Used in a Specialized Anti-Stalking Law Enforcement Unit', *Journal of Police and Criminal Psychology*, 26(2), pp. 128–142.

Sussex Police and Crime Commissioner (2021) Cyberstalking Increases Across Sussex in COVID-19. Available at: https://www.sussex-pcc.gov.uk/about/news/cyberstalking-increases-across-sussex-in-covid-19-crisis/

Sweeting, F., Arabaci-Hills, P. and Cole, T. (2021) 'Outcomes of Police Sexual Misconduct in the UK', *Policing A Journal of Policy and Practice*, 15(2), pp. 1339–1351.

SWGFL Safe, Secure, Online (2021) Revenge Porn Helpline and SWGfL Announce the Launch of StopNCII.org. Available at: https://swgfl.org.uk/magazine/revenge-porn-helpline-and-swgfl-announce-the-launch-of-stopncii-org/

Taylor-Dunn, H., Bowen, E. and Gilchrist, E. A. (2021) 'Reporting harassment and stalking to the police: A qualitative study of victims' experiences', *Journal of Interpersonal Violence*, 36 (11–12), pp. 5965–5992.

The Protection from Harassment Act. (1997) *The Protection from Harassment Act.* Available at: https://www.legislation.gov.uk/ukpga/1997/40/contents

The Sex Discrimination Act (SDA) (1986) Legislation, the Sex Discrimination Act 1986. Available at: https://onlinelibrary.wiley.com/doi/pdf/10.1111/j.1468-2230.1987.tb02589.x

Tjaden, P. G. (2009) 'Stalking policies and research in the United States: A twenty year retrospective', *European Journal on Criminal Policy and Research*, 15(3), pp. 261–278.

Trades Union Congress (2016) Still Just a Bit of Banter? Available at: https://www.tuc.org.uk/research-analysis/reports/still-just-bit-banter

Women's Aid (2021) What is Stalking? Available at: https://www.womensaid.org.uk/information-support/what-is-domestic-abuse/stalking/

YouGov (2017) Half of 18–24 Year-Old Women Say They've Been Sexually Harassed in a Public Place in Past 5 Years. Available at: https://yougov.co.uk/topics/lifestyle/articles-reports/2017/10/19/most-18-24-year-oldwomen-have-been-sexually-haras

YouGov (2018) Four in Ten Female Millennials Have Been Sent an Unsolicited Penis Photo. Available at: https://yougov.co.uk/topics/politics/articlesreports/2018/02/16/four-ten-female-millennials-been-sent-dick-pic

# 5   Trafficking of People for the Purpose of Sexual Exploitation

## Introduction

The World Health Organisation (2022) defines sexual exploitation as actual or attempted abuse of a position of vulnerability, differential power or trust, for sexual purposes, including, threatening or profiting monetarily, socially or politically from the sexual exploitation of another. Sexual exploitation can happen to men, women and children. It includes rape, forced prostitution, sexual photography, subjection to pornography or witnessing sexual acts and sexual assault or sexual acts to which the person is underage, or the adult who was pressured into or who has not consented. These sexual acts can happen in person or online. Many of the behaviours and literature on sexual exploitation have been covered in other chapters; this chapter will focus on human trafficking for sexual purposes.

Human trafficking is a form of slavery that involves the recruitment or movement of people for exploitation by the use of coercion, threat, force, fraud or the abuse of vulnerability (Gov.UK, 2022). It can occur when someone is trafficked across international borders or within the same country. For example, the UK is both a destination country for international trafficking and a source for its own national trafficking networks. The use of different recording methods and terminology for inclusion criteria means that estimates of the scale of the problem vary widely. The UK government last estimated 10,000–13,000 survivors of trafficking in the UK (Gov.UK, 2014), while these figures are now dated, they most likely underestimate the true prevalence of survivors in the UK (Cockbain and Bowers, 2019). Men, women and children may be trafficked for various purposes, including forced labour (for example, agriculture, food processing, manufacturing, car washing services), domestic servitude, forced begging and petty theft, and sexual exploitation. The most common forms of trafficking in the UK are forced labour and sex trafficking (Office for National Statistics [ONS], 2020).

Trafficking for sexual exploitation has become a major problem worldwide; a person can be sold multiple times by the same person, whereas a drug or firearm can only be sold once. This, therefore, means people are making a high-profit business out of sexual exploitation as people become 'durable' goods (Worden, 2018). It can often begin with a scheme of deception: a promise of good work in hospitality or modelling, or simply having a 'boyfriend'. The majority of survivors are women and adolescent girls; however, survivors of sex trafficking can be of any age and of either sex (Deshpande and Nour, 2013).

Once trafficked, survivors of sex trafficking often find themselves facing violence as a constant threat; they are particularly vulnerable to physical assault from traffickers, pimps, recruiters and customers (Gerassi, 2015). As a result, sex trafficking is a critical

DOI: 10.4324/9781003225461-5

health issue which requires both medical and legal attention. Health Care Practitioners (HCPs) in a clinical setting are ideally placed to aid identification, provide screening and offer assistance to survivors so they can access the services they require (Deshpande and Nour, 2013).

## Terminology and Definitions

The first internationally recognised definition of human trafficking was published in the UN and can be defined as follows: trafficking in persons shall mean the recruitment, transportation, transfer, harbouring or receipt of persons, by means of the threat or use of force or other forms of coercion, of abduction, of fraud, of deception, of abuse of power or of a position of vulnerability or of the giving or receiving of payments or benefits to achieve the consent of a person having control of another person, for the purpose of exploitation. Exploitation shall include, at a minimum, the exploitation of the prostitution of others or other forms of sexual exploitation, forced labour or services, slavery or practices similar to slavery, servitude or removal of organs (Palermo Protocol, 2000).

However, since this time there has been much debate in the literature around the 'transportation' of people who are trafficked and how this is defined, for example if someone can be a survivor of trafficking without crossing borders (Brayley and Cockbain, 2014). The most recent Modern Slavery Act (2015) in the UK does not imply that sex trafficking must include some form of travel or movement across borders, but rather that 'travel' can mean (a) arriving in, or entering, any country, (b) departing from any country and/or (c) travelling within any country. Sex trafficking is characterised by sexual exploitation through force, fraud or coercion.

'Sex trafficking' is a modern term (more traditionally it would have been called slavery) but the concept has existed for as long as we can account for, and with it, the abuse of power and human rights. The term 'sex trafficking' became popular during the women's rights movement in the 1980s, when female activists started protesting about the exploitation of women and girls in prostitution and pornography. Throughout the literature, there is most often, a distinguishing between prostitution/sex work and forced prostitution/sex trafficking. It is important to note that sex trafficking and prostitution are not synonymous. Sex trafficking often used as an overarching term used to describe commercial sex work such as prostitution, but also pornography, exotic dancing, stripping, live sex shows, mail-order brides, military prostitution and sexual tourism(Deshpande and Nour, 2013). Scholars argue that some women willingly enter sex work, albeit that it may be due to poverty and social circumstances, and others are forced or coerced (usually termed forced prostitution or sex trafficking). These distinctions are not always clear due to the variations in laws and lack of regulation around prostitution in most countries. For this reason, there are some schools of thought that question if prostitution is ever really a choice due to the persons economic or social background. They argue that the numbers of women who choose prostitution from a position of safety, equality and genuine alternatives are minimal (Moran and Farley, 2019). Whilst this debate is not one to be argued in this section, it is important to highlight due to the terminology you may come across in relation to prostitution/sex work and human trafficking. Furthermore, sometimes a person in forced prostitution can believe they are in a loving relationship with their pimp/boyfriend. They can be unaware that their consent to sex work may mean they are potentially being manipulated and coerced by a wider organisation. It is evident that there are complexities to these definitions; they can indeed be more 'grey' than 'black and white' which present difficulties for the individuals, society and legal frameworks alike.

## Background and Historical

It is important to note that human trafficking is not a new form of slavery; however, it is much more profitable today, than when the sale of human beings was conducted in open markets (Sigmon, 2008). Scholars such as Sigmon (2008) recognise the use of the newer term 'modern day slavery' and sometimes in the past century 'white slavery' to describe people exploitation of this generation. Some scholars differentiate between traditional slavery and 'modern day' slavery by identifying the move from master-slave relationship (i.e., legal ownership), to illegal control and forced labour.

In 2000, the USA passed the Trafficking Victims Protection Act (TVPA) and the United Nations the Palermo protocol (Protocol to Prevent, Suppress and Punish Trafficking in Persons, Especially Women and Children). Historically, however any focus on female survivors of sex trafficking had previously been associated with anti-prostitution campaigns (Alvarez and Alessi, 2012). One of the first prominent movements against sex trafficking in England was led by Josephine Butler, an English social reformer in the 1860s. She began a drive towards the abolition of child prostitution and fought for an end to trafficking of women and children into European prostitution. In the late 1860s she led a campaign to repeal the Contagious Diseases Acts. The Act brought about an attempt to control the spread of sexually transmitted diseases through the forced medical examination of prostitutes. Butlers campaign was successful and in 1886 there was a repeal of the Act (Jordan and Sharp, 2003). During this time, the was great focus on Europe, where survivors were primarily white, hence the term 'white slave trade'.

While such terms are now considered offensive, it is important to give context to the understanding of the legislation and language at the time. In 1904, the International Agreement for the Suppression of the White Slave Traffic was signed and in 1910 the International Convention for the Suppression of the White Slave Traffic (Allain, 2017). The convention stated: 'Whoever, in order to gratify the passions of another person, has procured, enticed, or led away, even with her consent, a woman or girl underage, for immoral purposes, shall be punished' A second article of the convention prohibited the use of fraud, violence, threats or abuse of authority to compel a woman or girl into 'immoral acts' (United Nations, 1951).

Josephine Butler went on to found the International Abolitionist Federation in 1875, with a focus on combatting sexual exploitation (Ray, 2006). However, it has since been argued that by associating human trafficking solely with prostitution, the conventions and international agreements that followed overlooked other types of labour and sexual exploitation, such as mail-bride arrangements or domestic servitude that came with an expectation of sexual favours (Ray, 2006).

During the world wars, the emphasis on such movements declined but by the 1960s there was resurgence in raising awareness surrounding the traffic of women and girls. By the 1970s, the violence against women (VAW) movement included human trafficking in its agenda with an emphasis on the violation of women's rights (Ray, 2006). At the same time however, there was a movement of those who called themselves 'sex workers';

they were opposed to seeing themselves as victims and thus wanted the right to redefine voluntary prostitution as sex work. As mentioned earlier, these distinctions are a source of much debate in the literature (Hussein, 2015), so whilst not argued in this book, they pose an important note when considering legislation surrounding sex work.

## Current Situation

It is estimated that there are over 5 million survivors of sex trafficking worldwide, of which children make up more than 20% (Toney-Butler, Ladd and Mittel, 2022). Statistics however vary; it is uncertain the scale of the problem due to the 'underground' nature of the crime. Furthermore, often statistics include all forms of trafficking making it difficult to know how many people are being trafficked solely for sexual purposes. Trafficking has become a rapidly growing global problem. From 2014 to 2016, the UK saw a 40% rise in the number of potential survivors of trafficking reported to local authorities and trafficking agencies (Lambine, 2018). When looking at adult sex trafficking specifically, the National Crime Agency (National Crime Agency [NCA], 2016) reported there were 880 reported sex trafficking survivors in 2016; the majority were from Albania (N = 391) followed by Nigeria (N = 95) and China (N = 50). The National Crime Agency (NCA) (2016) further states there was a 103% rise in child sex trafficking specifically from 2015 to 2016. At this time, the most common country of origin for child sex trafficking was within the UK, followed by Albania, Vietnam, Afghanistan and Eritrea.

Often, sex trafficking occurs through the exploitation of vulnerable people who are either economically or socially disadvantaged or both (Deshpande and Nour, 2013). People who are trafficked are often taken from less developed countries and transported to where they are deemed to be most 'profitable'. Sometimes people choose to leave their home country in search for a better life and end up at the hands of traffickers in the country they travel to (Hussein, 2015). Although debated in the literature, UK nationals can also be considered survivors of sex trafficking within the UK (Brayley and Cockbain, 2014); some statistics suggest that the most common nationality among children trafficked into and within the UK are British nationals (Serious Organised Crime Agency [SOCA], 2011). Traffickers need the people they are exploiting to be cooperative and therefore use different methods of control and intimidation, such as threats of violence to them or their family, drugging, removing documentation, debt bondage, preventing them from learning the language, isolation, moving the person from place to place and accommodating them in a way that they will become homeless if they leave (Marsh et al., 2012).

Furthermore, since the increased accessibility and use of digital platforms highlighted in Chapter 5, there has been a rise in cybersex trafficking. Flanagan (2022) defines cybersex trafficking as non-consensual cybersex between two or more people using a technologically mediated environment. Very often the person is exploited, and their abuse is streamed live on the internet via webcam, video, photography or other digital media (10Thousandwindows, 2021). Traffickers can be located anywhere in the world and can exploit people wherever there are means such as a tablet, phone, computer and internet access. Increasingly research has also indicated links between sex trafficking with social networking and online classified advertisements (Grubb, 2020). Increased knowledge and awareness of sex trafficking on these platforms has encouraged both the academic and private sectors to combat the crime through awareness, legislation and education, as well as through technological developments (Grubb, 2020; Giommoni and Ikwu, 2021).

Estimations of the extent of sex trafficking should be taken with caution. It is notoriously difficult to identify and track people who have been trafficked. Due to a variety of factors, survivors are often reluctant to report their situation, such as fear of traffickers and/or authorities, fear of deportation, language barriers, lack of education and intimidation (Lambine, 2018). Furthermore, in recent years the rise in the displacement of women and children due to the wars in Syria and Ukraine sadly poses an opportunity for traffickers to exploit people when they are at their most vulnerable (European Commission, 2022).

## Indicators People May Present with and Clinical Considerations

Survivors most often present with poor physical health, for example acute injuries, bacterial and other infections, burns, musculoskeletal injury, chronic physical pain, fatigue, exhaustion, poor nutrition, sexually transmitted infections, other sexual and reproductive health complications and unwanted pregnancy (Gov.UK, 2017). A literature review conducted by Hemmings et al. (2016) looking at survivor identification found that key indicators included signs of physical and sexual abuse, absence of documentation and being accompanied by a controlling companion. The majority of sex trafficking survivors report having depression, anxiety and/or posttraumatic stress disorder (PTSD) (Levine, 2017). In addition to these diagnoses, many survivors of sex trafficking experience self-harm, somatic complaints, aggressive behaviour, memory loss and cognitive problems, suicide ideation and secondary psychological issues such as alcohol and drug abuse (Oram et al., 2015; Levine, 2017). Furthermore, they might experience feelings of isolation, loneliness, shame, guilt, social withdrawal and risk of re-trafficking (Gov.uk, 2017).

Up to one in eight health professionals report previous contact with a person they knew or suspected had been trafficked (all forms of trafficking) (Ross et al., 2015). However, there is little evidence base to inform the identification, referral and care of trafficked people. Individuals who have experienced human trafficking encounter many barriers to primary care both during and after exploitation (Westwood et al., 2016; Williamson et al., 2020). A study that investigated access to and experiences of healthcare services in England for people who had been trafficked (30% reported being trafficked for sexual exploitation) found that respondents reported that traffickers restricted access to services, accompanied them or interpreted for them during consultations. Further barriers included requirements to present identity documents to register for care and poor access to interpreters (Westwood et al., 2016). Similarly, a qualitative study looking at health professionals' perceptions of barriers to care demonstrated that policies limiting entitlements to healthcare create significant obstacles to care, as do the inadequate resourcing of interpreter services, trafficking support services and specialist mental health services. In this study 'few healthcare professionals reported having received training on responses to trafficked people and most were unaware of support options and referral routes' (Westwood et al., 2016).

A study by Bick et al. (2017) looking at maternity care for women who had been trafficked showed that out of a sample of 98 women 29% reported one or more pregnancies while trafficked. Challenges that were acknowledged by both survivors and HCPs included 'restrictions placed on women's movements by traffickers, poor knowledge on how to access maternity care, poor understanding of healthcare entitlements and concerns about confidentiality'. Maternity care clinicians were able to recognise potential indicators of trafficking but suggested training would help them identify and respond to survivors.

## Impact of Sex Trafficking

### Individual

Individuals who have been sexually exploited through trafficking are likely to experience a multitude of physical and mental health problems. High levels of SVA are reported among women trafficked for sexual exploitation (Gov.UK, 2021). It obliterates lives by depriving individuals of their dignity, freedom and fundamental rights (European Commission, 2023). The following exert from a study conducted by Lederer and Wetzel (2014) who explored the health consequences of the survivors experience from sex trafficking demonstrates the sheer devastation.

> When I turned 13 I'd had enough of the abuse at home, and I ran away. I didn't know where to go so I went to the centre of town and stood by the town hall. A man saw me hanging around there and he said that he was looking for a 'protégé'. I didn't know what it was, but it sounded fine to me. He said I could stay at his house if I didn't have a place to stay…. When we got to his house, he pulled out a bottle of gin and had me drink and drink. The next thing I remember is waking up drunk in his bed all wet and hurt. He took me out on the street and told me what to do … During that time, I saw 10 to 20 men a day. I did what he said because he got violent when I sassed him. I took all kinds of drugs – even though I didn't really like most of them… Over the years I had pimps and customers who hit me, punched me, kicked me, beat me, slashed me with a razor. I had forced unprotected sex and got pregnant three times and had two abortions at [a clinic]. Afterward, I was back out on the street again. I have so many scars all over my body and so many injuries and so many illnesses. I have hepatitis C and stomach and back pain and a lot of psychological issues. I tried to commit suicide several times.
>
> (Kayla, Survivor)

Lederer and Wetzel (2014) state that this survivor's story represents '*not the worst that occurs in sex trafficking, but rather, the common experience of women and girls trafficked into commercial sex by a criminal industry*'. Similarly, to other types of sexual abuse and trauma, the impact is far reaching with adverse long-term affects noted. Studies suggest that individuals who have been survivors of trafficking may present with signs of emotional numbness, memory loss, anxiety and depression. There is also the likelihood that over time individuals may develop addictive behaviours in substance misuse or with alcohol, eating disorder and/or PTSD (Chon, 2021).

### The Wider Society

As suggested throughout this chapter, the sex trafficking of women and girls is an international problem. It impacts not just those who are being trafficked but also wider society in general. The crime as highlighted earlier brings high financial profits for those implicit in trafficking people. The trafficking of people is rarely carried out in isolation; very often it is interlinked with other forms of organised crime, such as drug trafficking, money laundering, extortion, fraud and property crime to name but a few (European Commission, 2023). The complexity of sex trafficking, arising from the vast criminal organisational structure, the underground nature of the phenomenon and the constant moving of survivors, reverberates throughout the world and poses far-reaching implications for wider society. From families to governments, the impact is felt culturally, emotionally, socially, politically and economically. The complex interplay undermines the security and safety of each, and every country involved.

## Current Legal Position and Policies Response

Although the legal definition of sex trafficking is now widely accepted, the debate over the nature of prostitution and therefore the laws and policies that apply to it are not straightforward. It is thought that the rapid growth in human trafficking is deemed by perpetrators to yield high profits with fairly low risks.

Prior to 2003, in the UK, there was a lack of specific legislation in relation to sex trafficking. Any suspected criminal cases were mostly dealt with as instances of kidnap or false imprisonment (Bartley, 2018). In 2003, the Sexual Offences Act criminalised trafficking, stipulating that trafficking for sexual exploitation would be classed as an offence in its own right and could attract a penalty of up to 14 years imprisonment. Included under the legislation was trafficking into, within or out of the UK. In 2004, all other forms of exploitation were criminalised under the Asylum and Immigration Act. Despite the legislation, in Britain, it was not until 2012 that the first people were convicted of child sex trafficking. The investigation into the Rochdale sex grooming gang exposed nine men who were subsequently convicted of numerous offences including that of sex trafficking. Currently in the UK, the Modern Slavery Act (2015) and the Human Trafficking and Exploitation (Scotland) Act (2015) effectively consolidate all existing offences of human trafficking and modern slavery, among these are bonded labour, withholding of travel documents and physical and/or sexual abuse. Tackling human trafficking and modern slavery continue to be one the main priorities within the National Crime Agency (NCA), more recently all efforts towards its eradication are led by the Modern Slavery Human Trafficking Unit (MSHTU). In recent years there has been an increase in investigations, prosecutions and convictions. The Office to Monitor and Combat Trafficking in Persons (2022) reported that the number of investigations had almost doubled with 3,335 cases in 2021 compared with 1,845 cases in 2020. In 2021, 466 defendants were prosecuted by the Crown Prosecution Service (CPS) with the courts then convicting 332 traffickers compared to 267 prosecutions and 197 convictions in the previous year (Office to Monitor and Combat Trafficking in Persons, 2022).

Nationally, there is a system currently in place for supporting survivors of human trafficking, namely the National Referral Mechanism (NRM). This referral system is available for certain professionals, such as NHS staff, police and those working in Local Authority to make a referral if they suspect an individual may be subject to trafficking. No consent to make the referral is required; however, it is advised that this is actioned and completed within 48 hours of disclosure. All referrals are sent to a Competent Authority who will scrutinise the referral form, with the intent for a decision to be made within the five working days. The Competent Authority resides in the UK Human

Trafficking Centre (UKHTC) which, from 2010, became a part of the Serious Organised Crime Agency. The UKHTC will assess all cases where the person being abused is British, an EEA national or in cases where there are no issues regarding immigration. By the end of 2018, the number of potential referrals for that year stood at 6,985 with almost a quarter (23%) of them being UK nationals (ONS, 2020).

For cases that hold links with immigration, the Competent Authority resides with the UK visas and immigration. These Competent Authorities have the power to grant all people who are trafficked with immigration issues a 45-day recovery period where the survivor is provided with safe accommodation, and support such as medical provision. During this time the survivor cannot be removed from the UK and a 'conclusive decision' will be made as to whether the individual is a survivor of trafficking (RightsofWomen, 2017). If the individual is recognised as a survivor of trafficking, the eligible recovery period is extended for up to one year and one day through the issuing of a residency permit. During this time, the survivor can appeal against any decisions surrounding immigration or asylum applications or they can at any point decide to return to the home country (RightsofWomen, 2017).

A recent report by the Office to Monitor and Combat Trafficking in Persons (2022), however, highlighted that despite the policy guidelines, there remain long waiting times for cases to be reviewed by the NMR and there remained inadequacies in the long-term care and support given following the review.

## Supporting the Individual

As highlighted earlier, explicit training for HCPs is limited yet studies in this area suggest that advocacy and assistance from HCPs are critical in the access to appropriate health services for people who have been trafficked (Westwood et al., 2016). Training to increase awareness and identify and helpfully respond to survivors of sex trafficking is needed alongside guidance on referral and support options and entitlements to care (Domoney et al., 2015). Williamson et al. (2020) suggest that improving access and use of healthcare services will require government interventions to ensure survivors are not denied healthcare.

Findings from a current literature review (Hemmings et al., 2016) highlighted the importance of interviewing possible survivors in private, using professional interpreters and building trust with the person. In order to build trust with survivors, the evidence suggests that health professionals should use 'sensitive, informal and non-judgmental language and acknowledge survivors' possible fears about the consequences of disclosing their experiences' (Hemmings et al., 2016). This review found that there is a need for a comprehensive needs assessment for people who have presented as a survivor of sex trafficking and indicate that they may need longer appointment times. It is suggested that HCPs adhere to principles of trauma-informed care, using open-ended questions (in order to reduce the risk of re-traumatisation) and demonstrating cultural sensitivity. More about supporting survivors is discussed in Chapter 10 (supporting survivors).

**Case Study 1**

Drita is an 18-year-old woman (Albanian Origin) who presents at Accident and Emergency with severe left-sided abdominal pain. She was dropped off by a man who claims to have found her on the street. She does not speak English very well and seems very afraid. She is sweating and looking very pale. She tests positive for pregnancy and an ultrasound reveals it is an ectopic pregnancy. You see bruises on her body, and she says she had a fall – she is reluctant to say very much, appears anxious, is constantly looking towards the door and wants to get out as soon as possible.

**How would you support Drita, what advice would you give?**

..........................................................................................................

..........................................................................................................

..........................................................................................................

..........................................................................................................

..........................................................................................................

..........................................................................................................

..........................................................................................................

..........................................................................................................

..........................................................................................................

..........................................................................................................

..........................................................................................................

..........................................................................................................

..........................................................................................................

..........................................................................................................

..........................................................................................................

..........................................................................................................

**Case Study 2**

Ana is a 23-year-old Polish woman who presents at the sexual health clinic with a male claiming to be her husband. Ana appears very nervous and seems to be holding the man's arm tightly. The man is reluctant to leave her side and wants to stay with her as he claims she cannot speak English. The man states that she wants to get tested for sexually transmitted infections as she has a rash on her labia. He explains it is painful for her when they have sex. He explains they are not registered with a GP and were hoping they could get antibiotics.

**How would you support Ana, what advice would you give?**

.......................................................................................................................

.......................................................................................................................

.......................................................................................................................

.......................................................................................................................

.......................................................................................................................

.......................................................................................................................

.......................................................................................................................

.......................................................................................................................

.......................................................................................................................

.......................................................................................................................

.......................................................................................................................

.......................................................................................................................

.......................................................................................................................

.......................................................................................................................

.......................................................................................................................

# References

Allain, J. (2017) 'White slave traffic in international law', *Journal of Trafficking and Human Exploitation*, 1(1), pp. 1–40.

Alvarez, M. B. and Alessi, E. J. (2012) 'Human trafficking is more than sex trafficking and prostitution: Implications for social work', *Affilia*, 27(2), pp. 142–152. https://doi.org/10.1177/0886109912443763

Bartley, L. V. (2018) 'Girl a: The truth about the Rochdale sex ring by the individual who stopped them: A CDA of a rape victim's testimony', *Applied Linguistics*, 39(3), pp. 352–372.

Bick, D., Howard, L. M., Oram, S. and Zimmerman, C. (2017) 'Maternity care for trafficked women: Survivor experiences and clinicians' perspectives in the United Kingdom's National Health Service', *Plos One*, 12(11). https://doi.org/10.1371/journal.pone.0187856.

Brayley, H. and Cockbain, E. (2014) 'British children can be trafficked too: Towards an inclusive definition of internal child sex trafficking', *Child Abuse Review*, 23(3), pp. 171–184.

Chon, K. (2021) *Mental Health Resources for Human Trafficking Survivors and Allies*. Administration for Children & Families. Available at: https://www.acf.hhs.gov/blog/2021/10/mental-health-resources-human-trafficking-survivors-and-allies#:~:text=Studies%20show%20that%20individuals%20who,%2C%20and%2For%20eating%20disorders.

Cockbain, E. and Bowers, K. (2019) 'Human trafficking for sex, labour and domestic servitude: How do key trafficking types compare and what are their predictors?', *Crime, Law and Social Change*, 72, pp. 9–34.

Deshpande, N. and Nour, N. (2013) 'Sex trafficking of women and girls', *Reviews in Obstetrics and Gynecology*, 6(1), pp. 22–7.

Domoney, J., Howard, L. M., Abas, M., Broadbent, M. and Oram, S. (2015) Mental health service responses to human trafficking: A qualitative study of professionals' experiences of providing care. *BMC Psychiatry*, https://doi.org/10.1186/s12888-015-0679-3.

European Commission (2022) Communication from the Commission to the European Parliament, the European Council, the Council, the European Economic and Social Committee and the Committee of the Regions on Welcoming those fleeing war in Ukraine: Readying Europe to meet the needs, COM/2022/131 final, available at https://ec.europa.eu/info/sites/default/files/communication_welcoming_those_fleeing_war_in_ukraine.pdf

European Commission (2023) *Together Against Trafficking in Human Beings*. Available at: https://home-affairs.ec.europa.eu/policies/internal-security/organised-crime-and-human-trafficking/together-against-trafficking-human-beings_en#:~:text=Trafficking%20in%20human%20beings%20is,committed%20by%20organised%20crime%20networks.

Flanagan, P. (2022) Cybersex Trafficking: The insidious side of the internet. In Essien, E.D. (2022) *Handbook of Research on Present and Future Paradigms in Human Trafficking*. Pennsylvania: IGI Global.

Gerassi, L. (2015) From exploitation to industry: Definitions, risks, and consequences of domestic sexual exploitation and sex work among women and girls. *Journal of Human Behavior in the Social Environment*, 25(6), pp. 591–605. https://doi.org/10.1080/10911359.2014.991055.

Giommoni, L. and Ikwu, R. (2021) Identifying human trafficking indicators in the UK online sex market. *Trends in Organised Crime*, https://doi.org/10.1007/s12117-021-09431-0.

Gov.UK. (2014) *Modern Slavery: An Application of Multiple Systems Estimation*. Available from: https://www.gov.uk/government/publications/modern-slavery-an-application-of-multiple-systems-estimation

Gov.UK. (2017) *Sexually Transmitted Infections (STIs): Migrant Health Guide*. Available from: https://www.gov.uk/guidance/sexually-transmitted-infections-stis-migrant-health-guide

Gov.UK. (2021) *Women's Health: Migrant Health Guide*. Available from: https://www.gov.uk/guidance/womens-health-migrant-health-guide#violence-against-women-and-girls

Gov.UK. (2022) *Human Trafficking: Migrant Health Guide*. Available from: https://www.gov.uk/guidance/human-trafficking-migrant-health-guide#full-publication-update-history

Grubb, J. A. (2020) The Rise of Sex Trafficking Online. *The Palgrave Handbook of International Cybercrime and Cyberdeviance*. pp. 1151–1175.

Hemmings, S., Jakobowitz, S., Abas, M., Bick, D., Howard, L. M., Stanley, N., Zimmerman, C. and Oram, S. (2016) 'Responding to the health needs of survivors of human trafficking: A systematic review', *BMC Health Services Research*, 29(16), p. 320. https://doi.org/10.1186/s12913-016-1538-8. PMID: 27473258; PMCID: PMC4966814.

Human Trafficking and Exploitation (Scotland) Act. (2015) *Acts of the Scottish Parliament*. Available from; https://www.legislation.gov.uk/asp/2015/12/contents/enacted

Hussein, R. A. (2015) 'The existing tensions in the defining of human trafficking at a UK and international level: A critical overview', *International Journal of Comparative and Applied Criminal Justice*, 39(2), pp. 129–138, https://doi.org/10.1080/01924036.2014.973051.

Jordan, J. and Sharp, I. (Eds.). (2003) *Josephine Butler and the Prostitution Campaigns* (Vols 1–5). Abingdon: Taylor & Francis. Available from: https://www.routledgehistoricalresources.com/feminism/sets/josephine-butler-and-the-prostitution-campaigns

Lambine, M. (2018) *Sex Trafficking in the UK: An Overview. Handbook of Sex Trafficking: Feminist Transnational Perspectives*, pp. 261–263.

Lederer, L. J. and Wetzel, C. A. (2014) 'The health consequences of sex trafficking and their implications for identifying victims in healthcare facilities', *Annals of Health Law*, 23, p. 61.

Levine, J. A. (2017) 'Mental health issues in survivors of sex trafficking', *Cogent Medicine*, 4(1), p. 1278841. https://doi.org/10.1080/2331205X.2017.1278841

Marsh, K., Sarmah, R., Davies, P., Froud, E., Mallender, J., Scalia, E., Munton, T., Zurawan, A., Powlton, L. and Tah, C. (2012) *An Evidence Assessment of the Routes of Human Trafficking into the UK*. Occasional paper, 103.

Modern Slavery Act (2015) *UK Public General Acts 2015 c.* Available from: https://www.legislation.gov.uk/ukpga/2015/30/section/2/enacted

Moran, R. and Farley, M. (2019) 'Consent, coercion, and culpability: Is prostitution stigmatized work or an exploitive and violent practice rooted in sex, race, and class inequality?, *Archives of Sexual Behavior*, 48(7), pp. 1947–1953.

National Crime Agency (NCA). (2016) *National Referral Mechanism Statistics – End of Year Summary 2016*. Available from; https://www.antislaverycommissioner.co.uk/media/1133/2016-nrm-end-of-year-summary.pdf

National Crime Agency (NCA) (2023) *Modern Slavery and Human Trafficking*. Available from: https://www.nationalcrimeagency.gov.uk/what-we-do/crime-threats/modern-slavery-and-human-trafficking

Office for National Statistics (ONS). (2020) *Modern Slavery in the UK: March 2020*. Available from: https://www.ons.gov.uk/peoplepopulationandcommunity/crimeandjustice/articles/modernslaveryintheuk/march2020

Office to Monitor and Combat Trafficking in Persons (2022) *2022 Trafficking in Persons Report: United Kingdom*. Available from: https://www.state.gov/reports/2022-trafficking-in-persons-report/united-kingdom/

Oram, S., Khondoker, M., Abas, M., Broadbent, M. and Howard, L. M. (2015) 'Characteristics of trafficked adults and children with severe mental illness: A historical cohort study', *The Lancet Psychiatry*, 2(12), pp. 1084–1091.

Palermo Protocol. (2000) UN General Assembly, Protocol to Prevent, Suppress and Punish Trafficking in Persons, Especially Women and Children, Supplementing the United Nations Convention against Transnational Organized Crime, 15 November 2000, available at: https://www.refworld.org/docid/4720706c0.html

Ray, N. (2006) 'Looking at trafficking through a new lens', *Cardozo JL & Gender*, 12, p. 909.

Rightsofwomen. (2017) *Trafficking and Modern Slavery*. Available from: https://rightsofwomen.org.uk/wp-content/uploads/2014/09/ROW_Trafficking-A4-DIGITAL-V2.pdf

Ross, C., Dimitrova, S., Howard, L. M., Dewey, M., Zimmerman, C. and Oram, S. (2015) 'Human trafficking and health: A cross-sectional survey of NHS professionals' contact with victims of human trafficking', *BMJ Open*, 5(8), p. e008682.

Serious Organised Crime Agency [SOCA]. (2011). *NRM Statistical Data April 2009 to June 2011.* National Referral Mechanism Data. Available from; https://assets.publishing.service.gov.uk/government/uploads/system/uploads/attachment_data/file/229080/0291.pdf

Sexual Offences Act (2003) *UK Public General Acts.* Available from; https://www.legislation.gov.uk/ukpga/2003/42/contents

Sigmon, J. N. (2008) 'Combating modern-day slavery: Issues in identifying and assisting victims of human trafficking worldwide', *Victims and Offenders*, 3(2–3), pp. 245–257.

The World Health Organisation. (2022) *Preventing and Responding to Sexual Exploitation, Abuse and Harassment.* Available from: https://www.who.int/initiatives/preventing-and-responding-to-sexual-exploitation-abuse-and-harassment#:~:text=Sexual%20exploitation%20is%20any%20actual,the%20sexual%20exploitation%20of%20another.

Toney-Butler, T. J., Ladd, M. and Mittel, O. (2022) *Human Trafficking.* StatPearls Publishing. Available from: https://www.ncbi.nlm.nih.gov/books/NBK430910/

United Nations. (1951) No. 1358. International convention' for the suppression of the white slave traffic, signed at Paris on 4 may 1910,' and as amended by the protocol signed at lake success, New York, 4 May 1949'. Available from: https://treaties.un.org/doc/Treaties/1951/08/19510814%2010-35%20PM/Ch_VII_9p.pdf

Westwood, J., Howard, L. M., Stanley, N., Zimmerman, C., Gerada, C. and Oram, S. (2016) Access to, and experiences of, healthcare services by trafficked people: Findings from a mixed-methods study in England. *British Journal of General Practice.* 66(652), pp. 794–801. https://doi.org/10.3399/bjgp16X687073. Epub 2016 Sep 26. PMID: 27672141; PMCID: PMC5072917.

Williamson, V., Borschmann, R., Zimmerman, C., Howard, L. M., Stanley, N. and Oram, S. (2020) Responding to the health needs of trafficked people: A qualitative study of professionals in England and Scotland. *Health & Social Care in the Community*, 28(1), pp. 173–181. https://doi.org/10.1111/hsc.12851.

Worden, D. (2018) 'Sex trafficking: Towards a human rights paradigm', *The International Journal of Human Rights*, 22(5), pp. 709–732.

# 6　Child Sexual Abuse

## Introduction

Whilst it is recognised that there are four overarching types of child abuse; physical, emotional, neglect and sexual abuse, this chapter will specifically look at child sexual abuse (CSA). That is not to say that if a child is subject to sexual abuse they do not suffer from neglect, physical and/or emotional abuse as they are very often interlinked. Episodes of CSA are diverse and complex; there can be contact whereby it happens in person or non-contact abuse where it happens online. UNICEF (2020) recognises a range of circumstances, whilst not exhaustive they state there are 'situations where a child is sexually abused by a relative or carer at home; raped by an intimate partner; made to or left with no option but to sell sex in exchange for food, cash or favours; sexually assaulted on the way to, or at, school by an adult, a gang or a peer living in the community; sexually abused by an adult in a position of trust or authority such as a pastor, police officer, care worker or sports coach; groomed or sexually exploited online by an adult or older child; trafficked within or across borders for the purpose of sexual exploitation, sometimes by organized groups of child sex offenders; or raped by a combatant or peacekeeper in the context of war, displacement or disaster' (p. 5).

CSA occurs worldwide, in every country and across all sections of society. It is a unique phenomenon and very often has dissimilar dynamics to that of the sexual abuse of adults. As a result, the way in which it is handled and managed differs from that of adult sexual abuse. In 2003, the World Health Organisation (WHO) identified a number of features that typify CSA; they include the following:

- Very rarely is physical force and/or violence used; in contrast the perpetrator uses manipulation to build the child's trust in order to hide the abuse.
- Typically, the perpetrator is a known and trusted caregiver.
- The occurrence of CSA spans many weeks or in some cases years.
- It is often a gradual process, whereby the perpetrator sexualises the child over time and as repeated episodes occur overtime, the more invasive they become.
- One third of all CSA cases are incest/intrafamilial abuse.

## Definitions and Terminology

Defining CSA is complex; worldwide there is yet to be a consensus on a definition or an interpretation of what constitutes 'child sexual abuse'. Even across the UK, there is no standard definition as each country's government defines CSA individually within their

DOI: 10.4324/9781003225461-6

own child protection guidelines (Gov.UK, 2018; Welsh Assembly Government, 2019; HM Government, 2021; Scottish Government, 2021).

However, despite the wording differences, the underlying premise of each definition is fundamentally the same, being derived from the WHO's definition formulated during the 1999 Consultation on Child Abuse Prevention.

'Child sexual abuse is the involvement of a child in sexual activity that he or she does not fully comprehend, is unable to give informed consent to, or for which the child is not developmentally prepared and cannot give consent, or that violates the laws or social taboos of society. CSA is evidenced by this activity between a child and an adult or another child who by age or development is in a relationship of responsibility, trust or power, the activity being intended to gratify or satisfy the needs of the other person. This may include but is not limited to:

- the inducement or coercion of a child to engage in any unlawful sexual activity.
- the exploitative use of a child in prostitution or other unlawful sexual practices.
- the exploitative use of children in pornographic performance and materials' (World Health Organisation [WHO], 2003).

As well as the lack of consensus of a worldwide definition, globally the terminology used also varies; umbrella terms such as 'child sexual abuse and exploitation' and 'sexual violence against children' are used interchangeably and incorporate the different acts of sexual abuse inclusive of the range of diverse relationships and settings. In addition, Mathews and Collin-Vezina (2019) identify multiple concepts being used which are both diverse and unclear in their meaning such as 'child sexual abuse, child sexual assault, child sexual victimization, child sexual exploitation, adverse sexual experiences, and unwanted sexual experiences' (p. 133). Within the UK, concepts such as unwanted sexual experience and child sexual exploitation, but not exhausted of, sit under the umbrella of 'child sexual abuse'.

## Historical Context in the UK

CSA is far from new and has existed for a long time. Historians have documented accounts from as far back as the 15th and 16th centuries (Mintz, 2012). From the 1880s CSA has been documented as a public concern and has been deemed to be a serious fault of the perpetrator or a crime. However, despite the rise in the age of consent from 13 to 16 in 1885 right up until post World War 1, there was little research or widespread public awareness, just the occasional criminal court prosecution of a sexual crime involving a minor (Bingham et al., 2016). Public beliefs werethat CSA was rare, it didn't happen to, by or within, ordinary loving families and that any reported incidences were focused on the lowest socio-economic groups. The possible factors for this are likely to be due to lack of understanding of lasting trauma, on the occasions when it was raised or prosecuted; the experts demonstrated more understanding to the perpetrator and large organisations that ran outside of public scrutiny, consistently denied and ignored the reality of CSA.

In the UK, up until 1960, CSA was considered under the umbrella of sexual offences inherited from the Victorian era, which predominantly focused on acts perpetrated by males on females or on the prohibition of any sexual acts between males. As such, age was rarely a primary consideration and was very often superseded by the gender of the parties involved. In 1960, the Indecency with Children Act came into power with it, brought the reference of children/child to be viewed as gender-neutral, enabling legal approaches to address the loopholes within existing laws. The Act also cited the offence to commit 'gross indecency' with or towards any child under 14 years of age or to incite them to such an act (Jackson, 2015).

Since the 1970s there has been an incomparable interest in the welfare of children and with this a notable growth in evidence surrounding the aetiology, prevalence and sequelae of CSA.

## Current Situation

The WHO (2020) estimates that globally in the past year, there are approximately 1 billion children aged between 2 and 17 who have experienced some form of sexual, physical or emotional abuse or neglect. Worldwide it is suggested that millions of children both girls and boys are subjected to some form of sexual abuse or exploitation. Of those children, it is estimated that 120 million girls have been forced to engage in sex or perform sexual acts before the age of 20 (UNICEF, 2020). The actual figures of CSA are unknown and, in reality, are likely to be much greater than estimated; findings from Stoltenborgh et al.'s (2011) review of 217 studies suggested that one in eight children worldwide had experienced sexual abuse before the age of 18 years.

Globally, it is recognised that CSA is gendered; the rate of reported sexual abuse is two to three times higher in girls than boys; however, in some nations or organisational settings such as same-sex residential establishments, the rates have been found to be higher for boys. Within most studies, 90% of the perpetrators are male (National Society for the Prevention of Cruelty to Children [NSPCC], 2021a,b). There are also developmental aspects; for younger children, very often the perpetrator is a family member or caregiver, whereas for older children there is greater exposure to a wider range of perpetrators, as well as family and neighbours, and they can be from positions of trust or of authority, peers and intimate partners. In the majority of episodes of CSA, the abuser is known to the child, with the child's or perpetrator's home being the most common location or where the abuse took place (NSPCC, 2021a,b).

As with the global prevalence, the UK actual figures of CSA are likely to be much higher than the reported statistics. Very often sexual abuse is hidden from view, under-identified as other adult members within a child's life may fail to recognise or confuse the signs of sexual abuse or the child themselves maybe too young, too ashamed, embarrassed or be too scared to speak out and tell someone. As a result, understanding the true prevalence is difficult to achieve and cannot be determined by a single set of reported figures alone. There are a number of different data sources that are reviewed in order to attempt to create a clearer picture of the scale and nature of CSA. Some of the data sources include police records of child sexual offences, children's services who identify children at risk, support services and adults who self-report about childhood experiences. A recent report by the National Society for the Prevention of Cruelty to Children (NSPCC) (2021a) estimated that '1 in 20' children in the UK have experienced sexual abuse, 90% of those abused knew the perpetrator and around a third of sexual abuse is carried out by other children. For those children known to children's services, either as subject to a child protection plan or who are on a child protection register, sexual abuse was identified in over 2,800 children nationally.

Over the five-year period (2015–2020), in the UK, the police reported a significant increase in the number of reported sexual offences against children (Office of National Statistics [ONS], 2020). Potential drivers for this increase include greater awareness of CSA by police in their recording processes and practices, the rise in investigations of historic CSA cases and the rise in technology with the internet making it easier for perpetrators to meet and abuse children. The current number of reported sexual offences against children for 2019/2020 is as follows: in England, under 16 years – 55,874; Scotland, under 16 years – 3,475; Wales, under 16 years – 1,881; and Northern Ireland, under 18 years – 1,517. The rates per 10,000 are 51.7, 51.2, 69.5 and 47.4, respectively. As highlighted in earlier chapters, it is estimated that less than a quarter of adults within England and Wales report sexual abuse, so it can be surmised that the actual number of child sexual offences recorded will also be significantly lower than what is actually happening. A noteworthy point is also that the police record the offences in the year they are reported not in the year they were committed; Office of National Statistics (ONS) (2020) figures for the year 2019 suggest that 34% of sexual offences against children occurred one year or more ago.

The Crime Survey for England and Wales [CSEW] Office of National Statistics (ONS), 2020) is a further avenue used to attempt to understand the rates of CSA by looking at adult's past experiences. It estimates that around 7.5% of the adult population (18–74 years) experienced sexual abuse under the age of 16 years – approximately 3.5% of men and 11.5% of women, with over a third being perpetrated by an acquaintance or friend. It is reported that approximately two thirds of reported CSA is intra-familial meaning it was perpetrated by a family member (McNeish and Scott, 2018). Many of the adults reported the main reason for non-disclosure at the time of the abuse was 'embarrassment'. Equally over a third of those who reported abuse experienced more than one type of sexual abuse and over half of those who were abused experienced or witnessed another type of abuse. For just over half (54%) of the adults who reported sexual abuse before the age of 16, the duration of the abuse lasted for less than one year, 25% reported the abuse occurred over a period of years between one and less than four. The duration of the abuse is also affected by the age of the child, when the abuse started, and difficulties associated with recalling the experiences. According to the global findings, women experienced multiple types of abuse compared to men (39% to 26%, respectively).

Support services have seen an increase in the number of incidences surrounding child sexual abuse; in 2019/2020 Childline counselling services dealt with 7,679 sessions about sexual abuse, and the NSPCC helpline responded to 8,612 contacts about sexual abuse: making them the ninth and fourth most discussed concern, respectively. In the same year, it was also one of the most common types of abuse reported by adults to the National Association for People Abused in Childhood's (NAPAC's) helpline.

## CSA within a Digital Context

As highlighted in Chapter 6, the last 20 years have seen an exponential increase in the use of technology, and the increased accessibility to digital platforms, digital services and digital information. As the UK holds one of the highest internet penetration rates across the world, it is inevitable that the children growing up in the UK have greater access and exposure to the digital world. Since 2018, it is suggested that as a result of increased social media and newer internet technologies, there has been an exponential growth in online offending (Gov.UK, 2021). Similarly, to the adult population, children can also become victims and in some cases find themselves perpetrators of technology-facilitated sexual violence (TFSV) (Henry and Powell, 2015, 2018). The overarching term TFSV includes an array of non-consensual digital sexual practices, such as image sharing, 'revenge porn', online sexual harassment, cyberbullying, 'slut shaming'.

As highlighted earlier, victims and survivors of CSA may be exposed to an array of different types of abuse. CSA, as discussed, can be initiated and executed by different perpetrators across a range of settings, and just as CSA can happen in person, it can also happen online. In 2020 the CSA Centre developed a document: a new typology of CSA offending. Within this document, CSA through 'online interaction' and through 'viewing, sharing and possessing images' is highlighted. 'CSA through online interaction' is defined as the type of abuse that focuses specifically on situations where a perpetrator, operating online, encourages/deceives/coerces a child or young person to take part in online sexualised conversations or sexual acts, and/or to produce images (photos or videos) of themselves which they share with the perpetrator online. This type does not involve contact abuse; where online sexual abuse leads to other types of abuse, this becomes an additional type of abuse (Centre of Expertise on Child Sexual Abuse, 2020, p. 15).

The connection between the victim and perpetrator is forged through the child or young person using the internet for the purpose of engaging in social and/or games purposes. The abuse takes place online through the use of digital platforms. The perpetrator can be a complete stranger situated anywhere in the world or they can be known to the victim, either as a family member, friend or acquaintance. The nature of the CSA may include a range of activity where the victim is deceived/coerced or encouraged to

- engage in conversations that are of a sexualised nature;
- initiate or take part in sexual activity online (either recorded or live);
- produce images;
- expose themselves whilst online via a webcam.

All of which may or may not include increasingly degrading acts. Likewise, the abuse may also involve the child receiving content of a sexualised nature (either recorded or live) by the perpetrator. Perpetrators of online CSA use specific approaches to reach their potential victims. They can use a 'scattergun approach' which aims to reach multiple children at any one time, or they can target an individual child or young person. Perpetrators may present as peers through either online gaming networks or social media making it difficult for their victims to recognise the risk. Perpetrators may use grooming techniques; they may initiate conversations that may quickly lead to sexualised content, normalise abuse through discussion, ask to move conversations/interactions to a private online space, convince the child or young person that they are in a relationship with them, send and/or encourage the sharing of sexualised images and/or threaten to share or expose images (Centre of Expertise on Child Sexual Abuse, 2020).

'CSA through viewing, sharing and possessing images' is defined by the Centre of Expertise on Child Sexual Abuse (2020) as the '*viewing of images of CSA that have already been created. This can include viewing, possessing and sharing images (photos or videos) with others, generally (but not exclusively) online*' (p. 16). This type of CSA is the sharing of digital but includes hard copy images (photos, videos and live streaming) of the abuse that has been taken place; the perpetrator isn't usually in direct contact with the child, but they are still abusing them by viewing the images shared by others. Acquiring and distributing images occurs over the open net and includes private messaging and the dark web. Along with depicting sexual abuse, very often the images also depict violence and other degrading acts; once they are made available, the speed of circulation across the networks makes it extremely difficult for them to be retrieved and removed (Centre of Expertise on Child Sexual Abuse, 2020).

Similar to CSA in person, CSA in a digital context is predominantly initiated and executed by perpetrators who are predominantly older than the child. However, recent studies have identified that children and young people especially those between 13 and 21 years are at an increased risk of exposure to unhealthy and upsetting behaviour within their peer group such as online sexual harassment, and image viewing/sharing (Project deSHAME, 2019; Setty, Ringrose and Regehr, 2023). Navigating the wide range of online platforms which include social networking services, communication and messaging services, and gaming and entertainment services, their capabilities and negotiating them for personal use is a complex process and online sexual abuse/harassment doesn't happen in isolation, it very often overlaps the online and offline worlds (Ringrose et al., 2012; Project deSHAME, 2019).

Project deSHAME (2019) refers to the umbrella term 'online sexual harassment' to encompass any unwanted sexual behaviour on any digital platform either public or private and includes non-consensual sharing of intimate images/videos, exploitation, threats or coercion, sexualised bullying and unwanted sexualisation. Unwanted sexual behaviour of any kind, in person or online, can make a child or young person feel frightened, scared, nervous, embarrassed, exploited, coerced and discriminated against. Recent studies suggest that young people hold an understanding of and can negotiate sexual consent from a physical perspective, yet they find navigating sexual consent in a digital context challenging (Ringrose et al., 2012; Setty, 2020a; Bragg et al., 2021). Whereas the Project deSHAME (2019) suggests that the understanding of young people, and consent surrounding sexual content, was more aligned with a 'digital empathy gap' (p. 36). Young people simply don't recognise the implications and consequences of posting and/or sharing sexual content due to a lack of education (Setty, 2020a, 2020b).

The digital empathy gap is more pronounced across genders. Within heteronormative relationships, studies suggest girls often feel pressurised by boys into sharing sexual body images, yet feel even if they share, their own wants and needs are not listened to or reciprocated (Ringrose et al., 2012; Setty, 2019). This contrasts with the reward and value experienced by boys for owning girls' images now coined by Hunehall Berndtsson and Odenbring (2021) as 'digital trophies' (p. 96). The showing and sharing of girls' body images in day-to-day life amongst young males is not recognised as abuse (Ringrose, Regehr and Whitehead, 2021). Meanwhile, unsolicited dick pics are normalised (Hayes and Dragiewicz, 2018; Ricciardelli and Adorjan, 2019). Indeed, Project deSHAME (2019) suggests that it is likely that many young people either experience or witness some kind of online sexual harassment. While it is acknowledged that some young people may in a consensual way generate images with age-appropriate peers, the future consequences are not always considered. It is suggested that even images produced consensually are shared without consent and therefore increasing the number of images/videos open to abuse from offenders. Gov.UK (2021) states that 44% of all CSA images reviewed and assessed by the Internet Watch Foundation (IWF) contained self-generated images or videos.

**Indicators People May Present with and Clinical Considerations**

One of the challenges of identifying CSA is, firstly, not all children realise they are being sexually abused, particularly if they are being groomed, but also for those who do, they may feel unable to come forward. According to the National Institute for Health and Care Excellence (2017), there are many barriers to disclosure. These include feeling confused, ashamed, guilty about the experience, as well as being afraid of stigma or blame or that they will not be believed. Children may also fear the repercussions of disclosure, which include fear that their family will split up; they may go into care or that the abuse may worsen. Some children who are experiencing sexual abuse care for their abuser and also worry about them getting into trouble. In view of this children may deny that they are experiencing abuse if asked. It is also important to recognise that some children may have communication difficulties or may not speak English fluently. Therefore, it is essential that the signs and indicators of CSA are communicated, not only to professionals but at societal level in order that we can all work together to safeguard children and that we acknowledge that abuse may be communicated indirectly through behaviour and appearance. What is also important to accept is that all children are vulnerable to abuse regardless of gender, ethnicity, background, sexuality or location. However, some are more vulnerable than others and this includes boys, children under the age of 10, girls between the ages of 15 and 17, LGBTQ children, BAME children, disabled young people and children who have experienced other forms of abuse. It is, therefore, important to be vigilant to signs of sexual abuse in all children.

The signs of CSA may be physical, behavioural and emotional and often a combination of these. Physical signs may include bruising, bleeding, discharge, pain or soreness in the genital or anal area, sexually transmitted infections. Pregnancy at a young age can also be an indicator of sexual abuse. Emotional and behavioural indicators include showing fear or avoidance of a particular person, nightmares or bed-wetting. Children experiencing sexual abuse may also allude to secrets or drop hints that abuse is happening without revealing it directly. Some children self-harm or develop eating problems or engage in alcohol or drug misuse as a behavioural response to the abuse they are experiencing. Some may present as withdrawn or aggressive, whereas some become clingier. Some children go missing from their home/placement. Displaying sexualised behaviour or having sexual knowledge that is inappropriate for the child's stage of development is also an indicator (NSPCC, 2021a,b). It is important to recognise any changes in behaviour, appearance, health, performance in school.

## Impact of CSA

### The Survivor

It is widely recognised that CSA has a significant impact on both the physical and emotional health and well-being of children and young people, which can have far-reaching consequences throughout adulthood. Being a survivor of CSA poses an increased risk of adverse outcomes; Fisher et al. (2017) identified seven areas that are impacted by the harm that is caused from CSA. Adverse outcomes can be in respect of their

- **Physical health** – possible long-term injuries, a high BMI, childbirth-related problems, and unexplained medical problems; gastrointestinal or gynaecological disorders.
- **Emotional well-being, mental health and internalising behaviours** – possible anxiety, depression, PTS, emotional distress, self-harm.
- **Externalising behaviours** – risky behaviours such as substance misuse, inappropriate sexual behaviours and offending.
- **Interpersonal relationships** – problems with intimacy, and parent/child relationships, poor relationship stability and/or satisfaction.
- **Socio-economic** – lower educational attainment (Mitchell, Becker-Blease and Soicher, 2021), unemployment, financial instability and possible homelessness.
- **Religious and spiritual beliefs** – using faith as a coping mechanism or a disillusion with religion.

- **Vulnerability to re-victimisation** – sexual re-victimisation in childhood and as an adult, other types of victimisations.

There is no linear pattern to these adverse outcomes, and neither is one experienced in isolation; there is often interaction between them meaning an adverse outcome may compound or mitigate other outcomes. The diverse and complex nature also means that there is no predictable time period for them to occur; they can occur or recur at any stage throughout the life course. Likewise, just because they haven't experienced a specific outcome at a specific time doesn't mean they won't at a later point in their lives.

Each survivor of CSA is an individual and as such the extent of the consequences they experience will differ significantly (Fisher et al., 2017). The impact of CSA is varied and attributable to a range of factors such as the types and severity of sexual offences experienced, the duration of the abuse, the developmental stage of the child and their level of understanding, their coping strategies and, lastly, the responses received from family, friends, community and services (Kendall-Tackett, 2008). Not all survivors of CSA will experience long-term harm; indeed there is evidence to suggest that some survivors exhibit resilience and/or achieve 'adaptive' or 'positive' functioning and recovery (Fisher et al., 2017). Similarly, to the adverse outcomes, resilience and recovery are not absolute; they are dynamic in nature and responses can fluctuate depending on their interaction with the social environment surrounding them. Disruption to resilience and recovery can be caused by the survivor of CSA being transported back to the abuse experience through (re)triggers of either a situation, event or sensation. Some common features include recounting the experience, specific sights, sound or smells, feelings of vulnerability or powerlessness and physical or sexual contact.

### The Family of Victims and Survivors

The disclosure of CSA has a direct impact on those surrounding the child. The perpetrator may be known to the family and as such the disclosure instantly changes the dynamic of all the relationships involved. Some family members/carers may be viewed as not being supportive or protective towards the victim in the initial period following disclosure; however, the majority become more so with time and support (Ullman, 2002; Lovett, 2004; van Toledo and Seymour, 2013; van Toledo and Seymour, 2016). Following a disclosure, it is widely reported that family members/carers experience an array of emotions, such as guilt, betrayal, powerlessness and uncertainties regarding investigations and the legal processes (Davies, Seymour and Read, 2001; Hill, 2001; van Toledo and Seymour, 2016; Barnardo's, 2023). Furthermore, the ramifications following disclosure may mean the loss of financial stability, familial and/or social support (Plummer and Eastin, 2007; van Toledo and Seymour, 2016) and possibly the re-emergence of historic CSA (Davies, Seymour and Read, 2001; Testa, Hoffman and Livingston, 2011).

Alongside their own emotions, is the uncertainty and/or difficulty of responding to, supporting and managing the needs of the victim, very often the child presents with changes to their behaviour such as withdrawal, aggression, sleep problems, addiction, sexualised behaviours or a mixture of them (van Toledo and Seymour, 2016). Studies suggest that the explanations, support and interventions received by the family member/carer are pivotal to them being able to provide safety and effective support to the victim (Miller and Dwyer, 1997; Jinich and Litrownik, 1999; Davies, Seymour and Read, 2001; Forbes et al., 2003; van Toledo and Seymour, 2016; Barnardo's, 2023).

*The Wider Society*

The ramifications of CSA to wider society are far reaching. CSA does not just affect those in the poorest communities but permeates all gender, racial, cultural and socio-economic boundaries (Anderson, Mangels and Langsam, 2004; McNeish and Scott, 2018). Synonymous with all types of Sexual Violence and Abuse (SVA), the effects of CSA carry a multitude of unseen costs. There are human emotional and physical costs placed on the survivor and family members/carers and financial costs which are placed on healthcare and support services, policing and judicial system and missed days at work which can impact employment productivity (Anderson, Mangels and Langsam, 2004; NSPCC, 2014). It is estimated that the overall cost attributed to CSA for 2018/2019 is £10.1 billion; nearly two thirds of the total are as a result of the human cost and their lost output (Gov.UK, 2021). Costs in anticipation (training costs) account for £7.8 million; costs as a consequence account for £6,709.6 million with the remaining £3,379.7 million used against responding to CSA (Gov.UK, 2021).

## Current Legal Position and Policies Response

The UK has signed up to the United Nations Convention on the Rights of the Child (United Nations Human Rights Office of the High Commissioner, 1989) and the European Convention on Human Rights (ECHR) (Council of Europe, 1950), both of which set out a number of rights for children. These include the rights of every child in the world to survive, grow, participate and fulfil their potential, be free from slavery, torture and cruel treatment. Additionally, these agreements set out standards of education, healthcare, social services and legislation and established the right of children to have a say in decisions that affect them. The UK signed up to the convention, and in 1989 the Human Rights Act made most of the ECHR UK law, and across the UK, the rights of children are included in legislation and policymaking. The rights of children in the UK were supported further by the Children Act (1989), which outlined key legal responsibilities concerning the welfare and safeguarding of children. This Act underpins the current child protection system today and outlines key principles, including the concept of parental responsibility, the paramount nature of the child's welfare and that children are best looked after by their family unless intervention in family life is essential. The latter Children Act (2004) placed a duty on local authorities in England to make arrangements to promote co-operation with key partners and local agencies with a view to improve the well-being of, safeguard and promote the welfare of, children when carrying out their functions. Under this Act the role of the Children's Commissioner was established to represent the views, interests and rights of children in policies or decisions affecting their lives. The Office of the Children's Commissioner is an executive non-departmental public body, sponsored by the Department for Education. The Safeguarding Vulnerable Groups Act (2006) was introduced to prevent those who are deemed unsuitable to work with children and young people being able to access them through workplaces. The Care Act of 2014, whilst principally aimed at adults, does also apply to children and young people. The Act enables decisions to be made in the child's best interest and is underpinned by the principles of empowerment, prevention, proportionality, protection, partnership and accountability. In 2017, the Children and Social Work Act was intended to improve care provision and support for looked after children. GDPR and Data Protection Act (2018) and the Information Sharing: Advice for Practitioners (HM Government, 2018) provide clear guidance, and surrounding information sharing and disclosure, the later developed to address the poor information sharing highlighted in a number of serious case reviews.

In support of the Act, there have been a number of policy guidance produced to guide organisations, agencies, staff and the public about safeguarding children and young people. Current policies include National Institute for Health and Care Excellence (2017) Child abuse and neglect; Working Together to Safeguard Children (Gov.UK, 2018; updated 2022); Sexual Violence and Sexual Harassment Between Children in Schools and Colleges (Department of Education, 2018); NSPCC CASPAR briefing (2018); Safeguarding Children and Young People: Roles and Competencies for Healthcare Staff (Royal College of Nursing, 2019); Keeping children safe in education (Gov.UK, 2022a,b). All of which emphasise the need for collaborative inter-agency working with clear communication pathways.

## Supporting Victims and Survivors

If someone presents in the healthcare system and discloses historical CSA, or a recent episode of CSA, it is important that this is taken seriously and in line with the correct system policies and protocols. It is important that time is taken by the HCP to listen to the persons' disclosure and respond with the appropriate tone and information. This is discussed further in Chapter 10 (supporting survivors).

## Specific Organisations Available to Signpost for Help and Support

Barnado's https://www.barnardos.org.uk/what-we-do/protecting-children/sexual-abuse
Childline https://www.childline.org.uk/
Parents protect https://www.parentsprotect.co.uk/services-for-survivors.htm
National Association for People Abused in Childhood https://napac.org.uk/
National Society for the Prevention of Cruelty to Children (NSPCC) https://www.nspcc.org.uk/
Safeline https://safeline.org.uk/support-for-family-friends/
The Samaritans https://www.samaritans.org/
Stop it now! UK and Ireland https://www.stopitnow.org.uk/

## Further Information

Below is a list of other documents that might be of use and inform your practice.
Children's Commissioner: https://www.childrenscommissioner.gov.uk/
Take some time to search the following papers.

- Protecting Children from Harm (Children's Commissioner) – A critical assessment of CSA in the family network in England and priorities for action.
- Preventing CSA: The role of schools – examines the important role schools can play in enabling children to recognise abuse.
- Investigating CSA – examines timescales for sexual abuse prosecutions and makes recommendations.

Centre for Expertise on CSA https://www.csacentre.org.uk/
Crown Prosecution Service – https://www.cps.gov.uk/

- Therapy: Provision of Therapy for Child Witnesses Prior to a Criminal Trial (CPS).

## Case Study 1

Aiysha (15 years old) has recently been contacted by Daniel (21 years old) by a private message via social media; he said he was a friend of one of her classmates and saw her on Aiysha's classmate's account.
Aiysha states, since the first contact, she and Daniel chat online every day. They like the same music, and he often sends her the sexy lyrics from the songs. Daniel persuaded her to send him 'Booby' pics and he sent her pictures of his penis. Aiysha feels he is her 'soulmate' and she believes they can have some sort of romantic relationship. Aiysha's friend accidentally sees one of the images on Aiysha's phone and confronts Aiysha about it.

**How would you support Aiysha, what advice would you give? What is your responsibility?**

........................................................................................................................

........................................................................................................................

........................................................................................................................

........................................................................................................................

........................................................................................................................

........................................................................................................................

........................................................................................................................

........................................................................................................................

........................................................................................................................

........................................................................................................................

........................................................................................................................

........................................................................................................................

........................................................................................................................

........................................................................................................................

........................................................................................................................

**Case Study 2**

As a child, Janice used to go stay with her grandfather when her mother worked nights. When she was eight years old, her grandfather started to come into her bed when he was babysitting. He did this for about four years. He used to touch her between her legs and make her touch his penis. As she got older, he used to make her watch videos and then coerce her to perform oral sex. Janice's grandfather recently passed away, and at the age of 26, she feels she can finally tell someone about what had happened to her as a child.

**How would you support Janice, what advice would you give? What is your responsibility?**

.................................................................................................................................

.................................................................................................................................

.................................................................................................................................

.................................................................................................................................

.................................................................................................................................

.................................................................................................................................

.................................................................................................................................

.................................................................................................................................

.................................................................................................................................

.................................................................................................................................

.................................................................................................................................

.................................................................................................................................

.................................................................................................................................

.................................................................................................................................

.................................................................................................................................

.................................................................................................................................

**Case Study 3**

Monika is 13 years old and went for a sleepover at her best friend Lou's house. Lou's stepdad was home from working away, everyone liked him, and all the girls thought he was attractive. When Monika went downstairs to get a drink, Lou's stepdad raped her. He kept saying he fancied her, and she must never tell anyone. Monika returned to the sleepover and tried to hide herself from the others. She called her mum to come and collect her first thing in the morning and she never went downstairs again until her mum arrived at the house. As soon as Monika got in the car, she burst into tears and told her mum what had happened.

**How would you support Monika and her mother, what advice would you give? What is your responsibility?**

..........................................................................................................................

..........................................................................................................................

..........................................................................................................................

..........................................................................................................................

..........................................................................................................................

..........................................................................................................................

..........................................................................................................................

..........................................................................................................................

..........................................................................................................................

..........................................................................................................................

..........................................................................................................................

..........................................................................................................................

..........................................................................................................................

..........................................................................................................................

..........................................................................................................................

# References

Anderson, J. F., Mangels, N. J. and Langsam, A. (2004) 'Child sexual abuse: A public health issue', *Criminal Justice Studies*, 17(1), pp. 107–126.

Barnardo's (2023) Child Sexual Abuse. Available at: https://www.barnardos.org.uk/what-we-do/protecting-children/sexual-abuse

Bingham, A., Delap, L., Jackson, L. and Settle, L. (2016) 'Historical child sexual abuse in England and Wales: The role for historians', *Journal of the History of Education Society*, 45(4), pp. 411–429.

Bragg, S., Ponsford, R., Meiksin, R., Emmerson, L. and Bonell, C. (2021) 'Dilemmas of school-based relationships and sexuality education for and about consent', *Sex Education*, 21(3), pp. 269–283.

Care Act (2014) Available at: https://www.legislation.gov.uk/ukpga/2014/23/contents/enacted

Centre of Expertise on Child Sexual Abuse (2020) A New Typology of Child Sexual Abuse Offending. Available at: https://www.csacentre.org.uk/documents/new-typology-of-child-sexual-abuse-offending/

Children Act (1989) Available at: https://www.legislation.gov.uk/ukpga/1989/41/contents

Children Act (2004) Available at: https://www.legislation.gov.uk/ukpga/2004/31/contents

Council of Europe (1950) European Convention on Human Rights as amended by Protocols Nos 11, 14 and 15. Supplemented by Protocols Nos 1, 4, 6, 7, 12, 13 and 16. Available at: https://www.echr.coe.int/Documents/Convention_ENG.pdf

Data Protection Act (2018) Available at: https://www.gov.uk/data-protection

Davies, E., Seymour, F. and Read, J. (2001) 'Children's and primary caretakers' perceptions of the sexual abuse investigation process: A New Zealand example', *Journal of Child Sexual Abuse*, 9, pp. 41–56.

Department of Education (2018) Sexual Violence and Sexual Harassment Between Children in Schools and Colleges Available at: https://www.gov.uk/government/publications/sexual-violence-and-sexual-harassment-between-children-in-schools-and-colleges

Fisher, C., Goldsmith, A., Hurcombe, R. and Soares, C. (2017) The Impacts of Child Sexual Abuse: A Rapid Evidence Assessment. Independent Inquiry into Child Sexual Abuse. https://www.iicsa.org.uk/reports-recommendations/publications/research/impacts-csa

Forbes, F., Duffy, J. C., Mok, J. and Lemvig, J. (2003) 'Early intervention service for non-abusing parents of victims of child sexual abuse', *British Journal of Psychiatry*, 183, pp. 66–72.

Gov.UK (2018) Working Together to Safeguard Children. Available at: https://www.gov.uk/government/publications/working-together-to-safeguard-children--2

Gov.UK (2021) The Economic and Social Cost of Contact Child Sexual Abuse. Available at: https://www.gov.uk/government/publications/the-economic-and-social-cost-of-contact-child-sexual-abuse/the-economic-and-social-cost-of-contact-child-sexual-abuse

Gov.UK (2022a) Keeping Children Safe in Education. Available at: https://consult.education.gov.uk/safeguarding-in-schools-team/kcsie-proposed-revisions-2022/supporting_documents/KCSIE%202022%20for%20consultation%20110122.pdf

Gov.UK. (2022b) Links to Legislation, Regulations and Statutory Guidance. Available at: https://www.gov.uk/government/publications/inspecting-local-authority-childrens-services-from-2018/links-to-legislation-regulations-and-statutory-guidance

Hayes, R. M. and Dragiewicz, M. (2018) 'Unsolicited dick pics: Erotica, exhibitionism or entitlement?', *Women's Studies International Forum*, 71, pp. 114–120.

Henry, N. and Powell, A. (2015) 'Technology-facilitated sexual violence and harassment against women', *Australia and New Zealand Journal of Criminology*, 448(1), pp. 104–118.

Henry, N. and Powell, A. (2018) 'Technology-facilitated sexual violence: A literature review of empirical research', *Trauma, Violence and Abuse*, 19(2), pp. 195–208.

Hill, A. (2001) '"No-one else could understand": Women's experiences of a support group run by and for mothers of sexually abused children', *British Journal of Social Work*, 31, pp. 385–397.

HM Government (2018) Information sharing Advice for practitioners providing safeguarding services to children, young people, parents and carers. Available at: https://assets.publishing.service. gov.uk/media/623c57d28fa8f540eea34c27/Information_sharing_advice_practitioners_ safeguarding_services.pdf

HM Government (2021) Tackling Child Sexual Abuse Strategy. Available at: https://assets. publishing.service.gov.uk/media/605c82328fa8f545dca2c643/Tackling_Child_Sexual_Abuse_ Strategy_2021.pdf

Hunehall Berndtsson, K. and Odenbring, Y. (2021) 'They don't even think about what the girl might think about it: students' views on sexting, gender inequalities and power realtins in school', *Journal of Gender Studies*, 30(1), pp. 91–101.

Jackson, L. A. (2015) 'Child Sexual Abuse in England and Wales: Prosecution and Prevalence', *History & Policy*, Available at: http://www.historyandpolicy.org/policy-papers/papers/ child-sexual-abuse-in-england-and-wales-prosecution-and-prevalence-1918-1970

Jinich, S. and Litrownik, A. J. (1999) 'Coping with sexual abuse: Development and evaluation of a videotape intervention for nonoffending parents', *Child Abuse & Neglect*, 23, pp. 175–190.

Kendall-Tackett, K. (2008) "Developmental Impact". In Finkelhor D. (Ed.), *Childhood Victimization*, Oxford: Oxford University Press.

Lovett, B. B. (2004) 'Child sexual abuse disclosure: Maternal response and other variable impacting the victim', *Child and Adolescent Social Work Journal*, 21, pp. 355–371.

Mathews, B. and Collin-Vezina, D. (2019) 'Child sexual abuse: Toward a conceptual model and definition', *Trauma, Violence & Abuse*, 20(2), pp. 131–148.

McNeish, D. and Scott, S. (2018) Key Messages from Research on Intra-Familial Child Sexual Abuse. Centre of Expertise on Child Sexual Abuse. Available at: https://www.csacentre.org.uk/ resources/key-messages/intra-familial-csa/

Miller, R. and Dwyer, J. (1997) 'Reclaiming the mother-daughter relationship after sexual abuse', *Australian and New Zealand Journal of Family Therapy*, 18, pp. 194–202.

Mintz, S. (2012) Placing Childhood Sexual Abuse in Historical Perspective. Social Science Research Council Available online https://tif.ssrc.org/2012/07/13/placing-childhood-sexual-abuse-in-historical-perspective/

Mitchell, J. M., Becker-Blease, K. A. and Soicher, R. N. (2021) 'Child sexual abuse, academic functioning and educational outcomes in emerging adulthood', *Journal Of Child Sexual Abuse*, 30(3), pp. 278–297.

National Institute for Health and Care Excellence (2017) Child Abuse and Neglect. NICE Guideline [NG76] available at: https://www.nice.org.uk/guidance/ng76/chapter/Recommendations# recognising-child-abuse-and-neglect

National Society for the Prevention of Cruelty to Children (NSPCC). (2014) Estimating the Costs of Child Sexual Abuse in the UK. Available at: https://library.nspcc.org.uk/heritagescripts/hapi. dll/search2?searchterm0=c5160

National Society for the Prevention of Cruelty to Children (NSPCC) (2018) CASPAR Briefing: Sexual Violence and Sexual Harassment between Children in Schools and Colleges 2018 Guidance. Available at: https://learning.nspcc.org.uk/media/1540/sexual-violence-harassment-in-schools-guidance-2018-caspar-briefing.pdf

National Society for the Prevention of Cruelty to Children (NSPCC). (2021a) Statistics Briefing: Child Sexual Abuse https://learning.nspcc.org.uk/media/1710/statistics-briefing-child-sexual-abuse.pdf

National Society for the Prevention of Cruelty to Children (NSPCC) (2021b) Protecting Children from Sexual Abuse. Available at: https://learning.nspcc.org.uk/child-abuse-and-neglect/ child-sexual-abuse#heading-top

Northern Ireland (2021) Stopping Domestic and Sexual Violence and Abuse in Northern Ireland Strategy https://www.health-ni.gov.uk/publications/stopping-domestic-and-sexual-violence-and-abuse-northern-ireland-strategy

Office of National Statistics (ONS) (2020) Child Sexual Abuse in England and Wales: Year Ending March 2019 https://www.ons.gov.uk/peoplepopulationandcommunity/crimeandjustice/articles/childsexualabuseinenglandandwales/yearendingmarch2019

Plummer, C. A. and Eastin, J. A. (2007) 'System intervention problems in child sexual abuse investigations: The mother's perspective', *Journal of Interpersonal Violence*, 22, pp. 775–787.

Project deSHAME (2019) Project deSHAME. Online Sexual Harassment. Understand, Prevent and Respond. Available at: https://hwb.gov.wales/api/storage/b51d7fc2-49e2-4b01-ade4-12b05b64daec/Handbook_Senior_Management_WALES_Print%20-%20English.pdf

Ricciardelli, R. and Adorjan, M. (2019) "If a girl's photo gets sent around, that's a way bigger deal that if a guy's photo gets sent around': Gender, sexting and the teenage years', *Journal of Gender Studies*, 28(5), pp. 563–577.

Ringrose, J., Gill, R., Livingstone, S. and Harvey, L. (2012) A Qualitative Study of Children, Young People and 'sexting': A Report Prepared for the NSPCC. Available at: https://eprints.lse.ac.uk/44216/1/__Libfile_repository_Content_Livingstone%2C%20S_A%20qualitative%20study%20of%20children%2C%20young%20people%20and%20%27sexting%27%20%28LSE%20RO%29.pdf

Ringrose, J., Regehr, K. and Whitehead, S. (2021) "Wanna Trade?': Cisheteronormative homosocial masculinity and the normalisation of abuse in youth digital sexual image exchange', *Journal of Gender Studies*, 31(2), pp. 243–261.

Royal College of Nursing (2019) Safeguarding Children and Young People: Roles and Competencies for Healthcare Staff. Available at: https://www.rcn.org.uk/Professional-Development/publications/pub-007366

Safeguarding Vulnerable Groups Act (2006) Available at: https://www.legislation.gov.uk/ukpga/2006/47/pdfs/ukpga_20060047_en.pdf

Scottish government (2021) National Guidance for Child Protection in Scotland. Available at: https://www.gov.scot/publications/national-guidance-child-protection-scotland-2021-updated-2023/

Setty, E. (2019) 'Meanings of bodily and sexual expression in youth sexting culture: Young women's negotiation of gendered risks and harms', *Sex Roles*, 80(9), pp. 586–606.

Setty, E. (2020a). *Risk and Harm in Youth Sexting Culture: Young people's Perspectives*. Oxon: Routledge.

Setty, E. (2020b) "Confident' and @hot' or 'desperate' and 'cowardly'? Meanings of young men's sexting practices in youth sexting culture', *Journal of Youth Studies*, 23(5), pp. 561–577.

Setty, E., Ringrose, J. and Regehr, K. (2023) "Chapter 4: Digital Sexual Violence and the Gendered Constraints of Consent in Youth Image Sharing". In Horvath, M. A. H. and Brown, J. M. (Eds.), *Rape: Challenging Contemporary Thinking – 10 Years On*. Oxon: Taylor Francis Group.

Stoltenborgh, M., van Ijzendoorn, M., Euser, E. and Bakermans-Kranenburg, M. (2011) 'A global perspective on child sexual abuse: Meta-analysis of prevalence around the world', *Child Maltreatment*, 16(2), pp. 79–101.

Testa, M., Hoffman, J. H. and Livingston, J. A. (2011) 'Intergenerational transmission of sexual victimization vulnerability as mediated via parenting', *Child Abuse & Neglect*, 35, pp. 363–371.

Ullman, S. E. (2002) 'Social reactions to child sexual abuse disclosures: A critical review', *Journal of Child Sexual Abuse*, 12, pp. 89–121.

UNICEF (2020) Action to End Child Sexual Abuse and Exploitation https://www.unicef.org/documents/action-end-child-sexual-abuse-and-exploitation

United Nations Human Rights Office of the High Commissioner (1989) Convention on the Rights of the Child. Available at: https://www.ohchr.org/EN/ProfessionalInterest/Pages/CRC.aspx

van Toledo, A. and Seymour, F. (2013) 'Interventions for caregivers of children who disclose sexual abuse: A review', *Clinical Psychology Review*, 33, pp. 772–781.

van Toledo, A. and Seymour, F. (2016) 'Caregiver needs following disclosure of child sexual abuse', *Journal of Child Sexual Abuse*, 25(4), pp. 403–414.

Welsh Assembly Government (2019) National Action Plan Preventing and Responding to Child Sexual Abuse Working Together to Safeguard People. Available at: https://gov.wales/sites/default/files/publications/2019-07/national-action-plan-preventing-and-responding-to-child-sexual-abuse.pdf

World Health Organisation (WHO) (1999) Report of the Consultation on Child Abuse Prevention. Geneva.

World Health Organisation (WHO) (2003) Chapter 7: Child Sexual Abuse in Guidelines for Medico-Legal Care for Victims of Sexual Violence. Available online https://apps.who.int/iris/handle/10665/42788

World Health Organisation (WHO) (2020) Global Status Report on Preventing Violence Against Children  https://www.who.int/teams/social-determinants-of-health/violence-prevention/global-status-report-on-violence-against-children-2020

# 7 Sexual Violence and Abuse in Marginalised Communities

## Introduction

Before starting this chapter, we believe it is important to recognise that, whilst informative, this chapter only touches the surface of sexual violence and abuse (SVA) in marginalised communities. A whole book in itself would be needed to explore the implications on health. We hope it provides an insight into the impact SVA has on these communities and an awareness of a more specific specialised support that may be needed.

The endemic of SVA has been observed in a number of specific circumstances, most notably conflict zones, remote and marginalised communities, and religious and state institutions. This chapter has a specific focus on SVA within those communities, which is a global concern and poses a threat to individuals human rights as well as collective peace and security.

## Conflict-Related SVA

Within the international community and among scholars and practitioners, the term conflict-related sexual violence (CRSV) is now widely used having been introduced by the UN Security Council resolution 1325 in 2000 (Independent Commission for Aid Impact [ICAI], 2020). Over the past decade there is increasing agreement that whilst CSRV occurs in a unique environment produced by conflict; it is part of a much wider continuum of gender-based violence that, whilst also affecting boys and men, is primarily perpetrated against girls and women (ICAI, 2020).

Efforts to address CRSV are driven by recognition of the devastating mental, physical, emotional, social and economic consequences of this brutal experience for women, girls, men and boys who live in areas of conflict around the world. It is also known that substantial numbers of children continue to be born as a result of CRSV and that, along with the mothers who give birth to them, they too are significantly affected as a result (United Kingdom Government, 2021).

## Definitions and Terminology

CRSV refers to rape, sexual slavery, forced prostitution, forced pregnancy, forced termination of pregnancy, enforced sterilisation, forced marriage and any other forms of sexual violence of comparable gravity that is directly or indirectly linked to a conflict and may be perpetrated against women, men, girls or boys (United Nations, 2022). The Statute of the International Criminal Court includes rape and some other forms of sexual

DOI: 10.4324/9781003225461-7

violence in the list of war crimes and in the list of acts that constitute crimes against humanity (International Committee of The Red Cross, 2016).

What distinguishes CRSV from SVA is that it is perpetrated as a mechanism to use rape and other forms of SVA to punish groups of people based on certain characteristics such as ethnic or religious or regional identities, assumed loyalties to other armed groups as opposed to SVA that is perpetrated by spouses, relatives, acquaintances or strangers (Koos, 2017).

## Historical Context

As with SVA, there are references to CRSV in historic texts, including the Old Testament and in ancient Greek texts, although it is accepted that historical accounts are unreliable and do not reflect the full extent of CSRV. For example, Stachow (2020) refers to the lack of Western records of CRSV during the Christian crusades, whereas during the same period, there is documented evidence in Muslim accounts. Stachow indicates that there is more consistent documentation of CRSV from the 1440s onwards and notes that English military policies show records that it was considered a justifiable act of revenge during times of conflict.

In 2022, Pramila Patten, the Secretary-General's Special Representative working to end rape as a weapon of war, in a high-level debate, referred to CRSVV as human tragedy, which is one of war's oldest, most silenced and least condemned crimes. In this debate she asserted that the ongoing impunity associated with this crime serves to normalise violence and that prosecution is not only critical for survivors but also as a form of prevention, which can turn the culture of impunity towards a culture of deterrence.

Whilst CRSV has been overwhelmingly treated as an unfortunate side effect of war with an enduring narrative suggesting it is used as a weapon, tool or tactic of war, there is actually very little support for this.

## Current Situation

Throughout this book the difficulty in gathering accurate data regarding prevalence of SVA is underlined. This is particularly the case for CSRV, where robust data is largely non-existent. This is explained by factors such as the instability of the conflict zones, which makes research and data capture extremely difficult, as well as the multi-faceted reasons for survivors not reporting their experience, compounded by stigma, fear of reprisal and the generalised repression by armed groups and governments (ICAI, 2020). The ICAI (2020) notes that whilst studies are rare, those that exist have found it difficult to draw reliable conclusions and as a result official statistics are both sparse and likely to significantly fail to accurately capture the scale of CSRV. Often conflict-related violence against women and girls (VAWG) is assumed to refer only to sexual violence; however, whilst this is known to increase during conflict, it exists alongside other forms of violence. For example, that which is perpetrated by an intimate partner, harmful patriarchal practices, child, early and forced marriage, sexual exploitation and abuse and femicide (What Works, 2019).

Child, early and forced marriage are common in patriarchal cultures and are considered to be both harmful and a violation of human rights connected to gender inequality, unequal gender norms, poverty and barriers to education. Child or early marriage involves any marriage where at least one of the individuals, disproportionately females, is under 18 years of age. Forced marriages involve one or both parties not giving their full and free consent to the marriage. In societies where child, early and forced marriage are prevalent, children sometimes appear to accept the marriage; however, this is because they have little understanding of their options, or because they have been coerced or forced to agree (Birchall, 2020). In fragile or conflict-affected parts of the world, the causes of child, early and forced marriage are compounded by displacement, being out of school, poverty and food insecurity weakening of the law and strengthening of harmful social norms. Mahmood (2016) highlights that in some parts of the world, for example, the Kurdistan region of Iraq, the influx of displaced people from parts of Iraq and refugees from Syria, meant many families felt it was safer for their daughters to be married. Other reasons are driven by poverty where the dowry payments associated with child, early and forced marriage can help families deal with lack of resources and using the promise of daughters for marriage in exchange for support with basic needs and safe travel to escape conflict (Birchall, 2020).

## Causes and Drivers of CSRV

As outlined previously, CSRV belongs on a continuum of SVA and is connected to gender inequality and the disempowerment of girls and women. However, gender inequality cannot fully explain the cause of this crime. For example, Maddux and Labrosse (2018: 18) refer to Sierra Leone where more CSRV was perpetrated by an armed group whose members were from an ethnic group who held stronger social norms about gender equality than other armed groups in this region. Equally, they cite reports of female fighters being involved in about a quarter of incidents of gang rape during the Sierra Leone civil war. In the ICAI review (2020) there are references to several examples where gender inequality in the conflict zone and the country/region of origin of armed groups in that zone do not explain the rates of CRSV and there is great variation in both frequency and the forms of sexual violence across conflicts, armed groups within conflict and units within these armed groups. The UN High Commissioner for Human Rights has received reports of 124 acts of CRSV in Ukraine; again, this is largely assumed to be underreported (United Nations [UN], 2022).

In the absence of a single theory or cause of CRSV, it is important to consider how CSRV is perpetrated in specific countries and contexts to try to understand ways to address it and assess the basic typologies. The ICAI (2020) suggests this assessment should focus on trying to understand the following:

- Who are the individual perpetrators and survivors?
- Who are the groups/organised units to which these individuals belong?
- In what locations is the violence occurring?
- What types of acts of sexual violence are being perpetrated?
- What are the cultural/societal norms and values?
- What is the context of the civil strife in which the violence takes place?

It is suggested that through such an assessment, it will help understand why and how CRSV occurs. By gaining an understanding of these elements, practitioners will be able to support those seeking healthcare that may have experienced CRSV.

## Individual/Societal Level Factors

The drivers of violence begin at the societal level where inequitable gender norms in the presence of armed conflict are significant determinants of CSRV. At the community level, the acceptance of discriminatory gender roles, normalisation of VAWG, as well as the increase in female-headed families are drivers of CRSV. This is compounded by the breakdown in social connectedness, reduced levels of social support and importantly the breakdown of law, which produces an environment where there are both increased levels of criminality and increased impunity for perpetrators (What Works, 2019). In turn, often the other institutions that would offer protective factors or support to women and girls in these areas are impacted by conflict in terms of ability to respond but also sometimes being involved in perpetrating CRSV.

Interpersonal factors are also thought to impact and the presence of conflict can bring about additional pressure on relationships. In areas experiencing conflict, often the immense changes to how people live, work and survive can challenge pre-existing social norms. For example, in some parts of the world, increased poverty brought about by conflict has meant that women need to work in order to support their families. This can challenge traditional dominant ideas about the role of women and also threaten the traditional role of men in family and social life; thus, triggering violence and unrest (What Works, 2019). Alongside this, there are individual risks which increase the likelihood of experiencing SVA, which include socio-economic conditions such as levels of educational attainment, poverty, age and social isolation, as well as acceptance of VAWG as a norm (What Works, 2019).

Some claim that CRSV is a crime of opportunity, but this explanation is criticised for contributing to harmful social narratives that suggest men are unable to control their sexual urges. However, there is evidence that there are causes of CRSV at an individual level. For example, there are reported cases where individual combatants respond to frustration with their military role, specifically when the expectations of social respect, status and remuneration are not met by perpetrating sexual violence (ICAI, 2020). A study by Elbert et al. (2013) which focused on eastern Congolese combatants found that 54% of the sample cited frustration as a cause of their engagement in CRSV. The study also found that some combatants perpetrated SVA as a means of seeking revenge, often for the loss of their colleagues. In this way, at the individual level, CRSV operates as a form of retribution but one that is made possible by the climate of impunity brought about by conflict. In conflict situations there is a breakdown of social and political order and weakening of social norms, which produces opportunities to perpetrate such crimes but equally results in states having limited or no capacity to enforce order and provide good governance (Nagel, 2021). Arguably in some parts of the world where there has been long-term conflict, the impact of socio-economic pressures, displacement and the ongoing breakdown of law, as well as the normalisation of violence, are conflict-related factors that increase the occurrence of VAWG as well as CRSV (Women for Women International, 2017).

Some research suggests that CRSV is a practice that emerges through social interactions rather than individual desires or as a result of organisational policy of command (Nagel, 2021). Nagel makes reference to research that focuses on the emergence of sexual violence in military groups and outlines its use as a means of integrating new recruits, where the focus is often on engaging in rituals which underline masculinity and suppress emotions. For example, Cohen (2017) suggests that as a socialising method, carrying out SVA is effective and efficient at enabling perpetrators to bond quickly and even single acts of SVA can bring about lasting bonds. It is these lasting bonds that account for the continued use of SVA in areas where conflict is inactive. For example, Donnelly (2019) refers to the use of SVA to coerce locals as well as reward fighters among members of al-Shabab in Somalia. Here, consistent with Cohen's argument, there are long-lasting ties among group members, where sexual violence becomes a normalised part of their activity and is used as an ongoing mechanism to both maintain group members loyalty but also to suppress civilians through control of sexual and reproductive capital.

### CRSV as a Strategy/Military Objective

Whilst there is a high correlation between VAWGduring and after, as well as in the lead up to conflict, it must be accepted that the reasons behind CRSV are multi-faceted and complex. There is evidence that in societies where patriarchal gender norms and identities exist that CSRV is much more likely to occur (Women for Women International, 2017). Koos (2017) refers to scholarly literature that examines the use of CSRV as a weapon of war. Such explanations indicated that CRSV is used to strategically terrorise, control, displace and eliminate the civilian population by targeting women. It is thought to be embedded in social ideas about gender, whereby historically the defence of women has been considered a hallmark of masculinity. Where conquering soldiers' rape or harm women, this is thought to destroy any remaining illusions of power for the men on the defeated side (Koos, 2017). Equally, in studies that explore use of CRSV against men, this is commonly considered to connect to the goal of demoralising and emasculating the defeated. So, where militarised notions of masculinity are prevalent, there is a much higher risk of CSRV (Women for Women International, 2017).

Elbert et al. (2013) noted that more than one quarter of the combatants they spoke to indicated that violence against women occurred as a result of direct orders or commands. However, there is very little evidence that commands are given that order combatants to carry out SVA or that it is used in a coordinated way as a terrorising tactic or to fight governments (Nagel, 2021). Indeed, whilst it may be that CRSV has been ordered, many studies where this is considered have at the best anecdotal evidence. It is also suggested that as a strategic military strategy, mass rape and other forms of CRSV can be counter-productive, as this can produce feelings of revenge that may mobilise civilians against the perpetrating group (Koos, 2017).

### Impact of CRSV

CSRV is not specific to any era, culture or continent, and as mentioned previously is recognised as a crime against humanity producing significant and enduring consequences for those who experience it, including not only the women and girls who are most likely to be targeted but also families and communities who are often destroyed by its impact.

What is key in the literature review conducted by the ICAI (2020) is that they make a clear move away from using the term victim, which is a term used widely in policy and literature focused on CRSV and SVA. The ICAI (2020) also suggests that the word victim is problematic in that it negates the agency of survivors, reduces their resilience and risks re-victimising them by reducing their primary identity to a body on which violence has been perpetrated through the label of victim (ICAI, 2020).

Swaine (2017) produced a report for the United Nations Entity for Gender Equality and the Empowerment of Women (UN Women). Focusing on CSRV in Indonesia, Nepal, the Philippines and Timor-Leste, the report highlights patterns of CSRV, which include a failure to address the harm experienced during times of conflict, examples of CSRV being perpetrated by state and non-state individuals, including sexual slavery. Women were also captured and held in detention where they experienced forced stripping, sexual torture, threats, rape, gang rape and mutilation of sexual organs. Some women were forced into 'marriages' by soldiers and in some cases conceived and bore multiple children, often being later abandoned by the soldiers when they rotated to other areas. There are many examples of pregnant women also experiencing torture and sexual assault as well as women being forced to bring their children into detention who in some cases were subject to CSRV and/or witnessed the violation of their mothers.

Whilst the true extent of CSRV is not known, Swaine's (2017) report highlights some of the enduring consequences for the survivors. These are far reaching, and the impact cannot be overstated. Unwanted pregnancy or loss of existing pregnancy is common alongside physical pain from injuries and psychological harm and trauma. Survivors also report feelings of insecurity which is often a result of intimidation by perpetrators and fear of retaliation for reporting CRSV but also the insecurity brought about by actual and potential violence from their own family and community. In many cases survivors experience stigma and discrimination or rejection of their families and communities, which means they are socially excluded and isolated. This leads to marginalisation and increased vulnerability. To add to this the impunity associated with CRSV means that survivors often do not receive justice or reparation for the harm they and their children have experienced. For some women who have been forced into 'marriage' to soldiers, they face ongoing challenges in relation to dealing with a long-term association with the perpetrator, often compelled to remain with the abuser to remain with their children, given that in many patriarchal societies women do not hold primary legal claim to their children.

### Children Born as a Result of CRSV

Children who are born as a result of CRSV are estimated to be amongst the most at risk in war-affected populations, but Swaine (2017) highlights the lack of attention these children often receive. These children, along with their mothers, experience the loss of wider family support due to the exclusion of their mother, as well as experiencing the wider social stigma and discrimination. In many cases, they may be aware of or have witnessed the harm perpetrated towards their mother. Given the decline in policing protection and breakdown of the legal system in these areas, children are not well protected by statutory bodies and are at high risk of trafficking. Compounding this due to fragmented, weakened and overburdened function of protective organisations in areas of conflict, these children often do not receive the protection or support they need (Swaine, 2017).

It is accepted that there are long-term consequences for these children which are driven by social and cultural attitudes towards their mothers as survivors of CRSV and also concerning their birth origins. Sometimes these children face abandonment or are placed in institutions of care. Others do remain with their mothers or family but are often socially and economically marginalised. These children are at much greater risk of a multitude of negative physical and mental health impacts resulting from their experiences and are known to experience difficult relationships with their mothers and wider family, as well as feelings of guilt, shame, isolation and blame (Swaine, 2017).

Individuals who have experienced CRSV have specific and complex health needs due to the traumatic nature of their experiences. Here are some of the key health needs of survivors of CRSV to be aware of:

1 Physical health: Survivors may have physical injuries and health complications resulting from the SVA they experienced. These can include injuries, infections, sexually transmitted infections (STIs) and gynaecological issues.
2 Psychological and emotional support: Survivors often experience severe psychological trauma, including post-traumatic stress (PTS), depression, anxiety and other mental health issues. Access to mental health services, counselling and psychosocial support is crucial for their recovery and healing.
3 Reproductive health: Survivors may face unwanted pregnancies, unsafe abortions and reproductive health complications because of SVA. Access to reproductive health services, including family planning and safe abortion services where legal, is important for survivors to exercise control over their reproductive choices. Gynaecological support for any ongoing complication of injuries or experiences of female genital mutilation (FGM) will need to be considered.
4 Access to justice and legal support: Many survivors of CRSV face barriers in seeking justice and accountability for the crimes committed against them. Signposting to legal support, including help navigating the legal system and seeking redress, is essential.
5 Social support and reintegration: Survivors often experience stigmatisation and isolation within their communities. Support for integration or reintegration into communities, as well as addressing social and economic needs, can aid in their recovery and reduce the risk of further harm. It is important to consider the needs of those who have fled another country due to the violence, the specific support they will need should be addressed by social care, specialist organisations and voluntary organisational support.
6 Safety and security: Ensuring the safety and security of survivors is critical to protect them from further harm and to facilitate their access to necessary services.
7 Prevention of further violence: Efforts to prevent further instances of CRSV are crucial. For example, are there any trips back to the country the violence was perpetrated in booked?
8 Awareness and education: Promoting awareness and education about CRSV can help reduce stigma, improve access to services and foster a supportive environment for survivors.

Addressing the health needs of survivors of CRSV requires a multidisciplinary and coordinated approach involving healthcare providers, mental health professionals, legal experts, humanitarian organisations and the community at large. Empowering survivors to share their experiences and participate in decision-making processes can also contribute to their healing and overall well-being.

## Female Genital Mutilation

FGM is recognised as a violation of human rights and has serious physical and psychological consequences for the affected individuals. Also known as female genital cutting or female circumcision, FGM refers to the practice of partially or completely removing or altering the external female genitalia for non-medical reasons. It is a deeply rooted cultural and traditional practice that has been performed in some communities for centuries, usually in girls from infancy to 15 years. The World Health Organisation (WHO) (2023) state that FGM effects more than 200 million girls and women from 200 countries, largely; Africa, the Middle East and Asia. FGM exists within socio-cultural and social norms of those communities that practice it for numerous reasons, the most common being:

- Pressure to conform to social norms, families experiencing fear of being rejected by the community if they do not allow the practice to be undertaken on their girl(s).
- Considered a necessary part of raising a girl, to prepare for adulthood by controlling her sexuality to promote pre-marital virginity and fidelity. However, in many of those communities that participate in this practice SVA is the norm, therefore, putting the girl at more risk of injury in the future.

FGM has no health benefits. It involves removing and damaging healthy and normal female genital tissue. Complications of FGM can include as follows:

- severe pain
- excessive bleeding (haemorrhage)
- genital tissue swelling/damage to tissue
- fever
- infection/sepsis
- urinary problems
- death

Long-term complications can include as follows:

- urinary problems (painful urination, urinary tract infections);
- vaginal problems (discharge, itching, bacterial vaginosis and other infections);
- menstrual problems (painful menstruations, difficulty in passing menstrual blood etc.);
- scar tissue and keloid;
- sexual problems (pain during intercourse, decreased satisfaction etc.);
- increased risk of childbirth complications (difficult delivery, excessive bleeding, caesarean section, need to resuscitate the baby etc.) and newborn deaths;
- need for later surgeries: for example, the sealing or narrowing of the vaginal opening may lead to the practice of cutting open the sealed vagina later to allow for sexual intercourse and childbirth. Sometimes genital tissue is stitched again several times, including after childbirth, hence the woman goes through repeated opening and closing procedures, further increasing both immediate and long-term risks and
- psychological problems (depression, anxiety, PTS disorder, low self-esteem etc.).

(WHO, 2023)

In the UK, FGM is illegal (Home Office, 2023). It is an offence to perform FGM and to assist a person performing FGM on themselves. It is also illegal to facilitate FGM (whether performing or assisting) abroad on a UK national or UK resident. If you suspect FGM has or is about to take place, contact your organisations safeguarding lead and/or the local authority designated lead. Further guidance for UK practitioners can be found in Working Together to Safeguard Children (2018). If you think someone is in immediate danger, contact the police and the Foreign and Commonwealth Office (+44 020 70081500) if she's already been taken abroad. For those international practitioners, please search your regional and district safeguarding policies/procedures.

## Prevention of CSRV

Prevention of CRSV is complex and requires a multi-faceted approach to address entrenched political, social, economic, environmental and cultural drivers of conflict. However, it must be remembered that CSRV is not inevitable and through the right interventions and disincentives is entirely preventable. CRSV is often considered a direct expression of gender inequality and occurs in the context of other forms of gender-based violence, including sexual violence (United Nations Office of the Special Representative of the Secretary General on Sexual Violence in Conflict, [UNOSRSG], 2022). The prevention of CSRV contributes to the achievement of sustainable development goals by promoting gender equality, reducing social inequalities and promoting peace and justice internationally. The framework for the prevention of CRSV (UNOSRSG, 2022) focuses on prevention but also promotes a survivor-centred approach.

Addressing CRSV is both a UK and global priority, and whilst it is prohibited under international law, in 2021, incidents continued to be reported in 18 countries (United Kingdom Government, 2022). The Murad Code (2022) is a living document that is to be reviewed periodically. It is a voluntary, global code of conduct which outlines minimum standards for the safe, effective and ethical gathering and use of information relating to victims and/or survivors of CRSV. The code is embedded within international law and the human rights of those who have experienced CRSV to dignity, privacy, health, security and access to justice, truth, and an effective remedy. It applies to individuals as well as organisations and underlines the collective responsibility to work together to develop, maintain and improve survivor-centred practices.

The UK Department for International Development invested an unprecedented £25 million over five years to prevent VAWG, primarily focusing efforts on Africa and Asia. A flagship programme introduced from these funds: The What Works to Prevent Violence against Women and Girls Programme focuses on generating evidence from rigorous primary research and evaluations of exciting interventions to understand What Works to prevent VAWG generally, and also specifically in fragile and conflict areas. The component of the programme focused on VAWG in conflict and areas of humanitarian crises aims to conduct and disseminate rigorous research in this area in order to understand better the prevalence, forms, trends and drivers of VAWG, as well as to identify effective mechanisms to prevent and respond to it. One of the challenges of developing a robust evidence base is that in these areas those conducting such research face challenges in terms of ethics and safety.

## Sexual Violence and Abuse in Marginalised Communities

Many people who experience SVA are also faced with intersectional discrimination due to their gender, disabilities, ethnicity, sexual orientation and/or cultural identities. These people are at higher risk of abuse and even less likely to report their abuse to the authorities or healthcare providers. When talking about SVA and survivors, we need to be aware that minorities and any marginalised groups are often the most vulnerable and the ones who struggle the most to gain protection and helpful resources.

Marginalised populations are groups and communities that experience discrimination and exclusion because of unequal power relationships across economic, political, social and cultural dimensions (Sevelius et al., 2020). People in these communities are considered to be those who are disadvantaged, medically underserved or difficult to reach; they, therefore, are more likely to experience inequalities from a health and social care perspective. Examples of marginalised communities are racial/cultural minorities, the LGBTQ+ community, persons with cognitive or physical impairments, traveller communities and more.

## Prevalence

Statistics show that domestic abuse is a significant health issues for the travelling community, with an estimate that between 60% and 80% of women from these communities experience abuse compared to 25% of the female population generally (Doncaster Council, 2022). One in two bisexual women have experienced rape in their lifetime (Chen et al., 2020). James et al. (2016) estimate that between 47% and 58% of trans people have experienced SVA in their lifetime with that number jumping to 80% for those identifying as bi+ or non-binary (Flanders, Anderson and Tarasoff, 2020). Research has consistently identified higher rates of SVA among sexual minoritised people compared to heterosexual (Hughes et al., 2010; Chen et al., 2020; Flanders et al., 2023). These statistics are shockingly high and a reminder that as health practitioners, SVA discussion with these population is essential to ensuring their health needs are supported.

Survivors of SVA from marginalised communities often encounter additional barriers to seeking safety and receiving support. Below are just some of the barriers that survivors in these communities may experience:

- **Stereotypes:** Stereotypes aim to hypersexualise, objectify and dehumanise marginalised survivors. Stereotypes contribute to rape myth acceptance, therefore, often hindering belief and support.
- **Invisibility:** To maintain an oppressive status quo and misrepresentation, our society dismisses certain identities and issues. One example of this is the lack of gender-inclusive toilets, and exclusively using he/she pronouns creates additional barriers for these survivors. As a result, trans and non-binary voices may not be heard or respected or feel welcomed to use health services that are not inclusive. Alongside this, discrimination is often experienced when accessing health and social care services due to lack of knowledge and understanding of their needs from professionals involved in their care.
- **Fear of being outed:** The disclosure of an LGBTQ+ person's sexual orientation and/ or gender identity without their consent or feeling forced into a disclosure can have serious consequences, despite the Equality Act (2010). They may experience discrimination, physical violence and the denial of employment. In addition, they may be shunned, shamed and disowned by family, friends and houses of worship. The possibility of further victimisation and hardship only complicates the process of both disclosure of SVA and healing for many LGBTQ+ survivors.
- **Poverty/homelessness:** People in marginalised communities experience poverty (also from a health perspective) and homelessness at disproportionate rates. This is not a

coincidence, but another reflection of intersectionality and oppression in our society. Survivors living in these circumstances are often unable to afford legal or obtain/have accessible transportation necessary to receive treatment from healthcare providers. For example, trapped by culture, poor literacy and education, distrust of the police and social services, and fear of separation from family and friends, gypsy and traveller women are far less likely to report incidences of SVA or to seek help. Further, those with long-term health conditions or disabilities may not be able to divert time and energy away from meeting their basic survival needs.

- **Language and accessibility:** Survivors who don't speak English, or speak English as a second or other language, face a shortage of accessible resources. The lack of non-English services can include sexual assault nurse examinations (SANEs), case management, psychological support and legal advocacy. Helplines, which are usually relied on to connect survivors to services, may also be inaccessible. As a result, people can either fall through the cracks or feel 'othered' after being sent to an alternative service. In addition to language barriers, spaces (face to face or virtual) may also not be accessible in accommodating to survivors living with disabilities. Examples include antiquated SANE beds, lack of ramps and elevators, multiple appointments with a range of professionals and confidentiality mechanisms that exclude sharing information with personal care assistants. This may lead to survivors feeling invisible and insignificant, on top of not having their needs met.

When marginalised survivors are repeatedly exposed to the negative messages that have been cast against them, they begin to internalise their oppression (David, 2014). They may perpetuate roles and stereotypes that hypersexualise, objectify and dehumanise as a way of carrying out a self-fulfilling prophecy. For example, people who have been told they are over sexualising themselves on special media by society may not report SVA, as they are convinced it was somehow justified. Others may have normalised an abusive reality because they believe they are inferior and deserve the behaviour directed to them. All of these contribute not only to barriers for disclosure but also to accessing health services following disclosure. Therefore, a supportive and inclusive response from practitioners is essential.

## Ritual-Related Sexual Violence and Abuse

Ritual-related SVA is a controversial and highly debated topic. It refers to allegations or claims of sexual abuse occurring within the context of rituals or ceremonies, often associated with cults, secret societies or occult practices. Organised abuse within an ideological framework (that is a belief system sometimes including symbols or group activities with sometimes religious or supernatural connotations) is referred to as 'ritual abuse' (Salter, 2012). It is sometimes considered a strategic practice through which some organised groups indoctrinate children into a violently misogynistic worldview, to retain control over the victims and to exculpate acts of violence (Salter, 2012; Schroder et al., 2020). Research surrounding this topic overwhelmingly explores childhood experiences/reports of ritual abuse, therefore, please see Chapter 8 – Child Sex Abuse – to explore how to support survivors. These allegations may involve claims of organised, systematic and extreme forms of sexual abuse, which may include elements of sadism, torture and mind control. It's essential to note that the existence of ritual-related sexual abuse is a contentious issue within the fields of psychology, criminology and sociology.

In the past, there have been high-profile cases and moral panics related to satanic ritual abuse (SRA), which gained significant attention in the 1980s and early 1990s. However, subsequent investigations and research often found little evidence to support the existence of large, organised and widespread Satanic cults carrying out ritual abuse as described in some media reports. Health and mental health professionals need to handle these cases with care and objectivity, seeking specialist support from safeguarding leads.

In all of the experiences discussed above, it is essential that practitioners are aware and sensitive to people's backgrounds and fears of further violence/persecution. Understanding and respecting the differences in our communities are the first step to being able to provide appropriate and safe support for those who may be experiencing, or have experiences, SVA. Organisations that support these individuals are often very specific; familiarising yourself with those in your communities will aid in fostering growing relationship that can aid in survivors feeling heard and supported.

| Regional organisations providing support for marginalised communities | Their focus: (i.e., Black Minoritised Women and LGBTQ) |
|---|---|
|  |  |
|  |  |
|  |  |
|  |  |
|  |  |
|  |  |
|  |  |

## Additional and National Support Organisations

- https://www.sistahspace.org/ supporting African and Caribbean heritage women affected by domestic and sexual abuse.
- https://www.hersana.org/. providing Black femme survivors with support, access to justice and holistic therapies around all forms of gender-based violence.
- https://www.opoka.org.uk/. Opoka helps women and children in the Polish community to improve health, well-being, financial stability and happiness by stopping domestic violence.
- Imkaan is the only UK-based, umbrella women's organisation dedicated to addressing violence against Black and minoritised women and girls. They have an excellent resource for all national helplines that can aid most minoritised women and girls who have, or is, experiencing SVA: https://www.imkaan.org.uk/get-help

**Case Study 1**

Sarah is 16 years old. She is originally from Sudan. Her family moved to the region seven years ago. She is attending your clinical area with a suspected kidney infection. She suffers from long-term recurrent urinary tract infections; however, this has never been referred or investigated fully.

She has never been vaginally examined as she, and her parents, has always refused. She is attending alone for her appointment for the first time. She disclosed she is embarrassed to be examined as she is different 'down there' (meaning vaginally) because of being 'cut'. She asks you not to tell anyone.

- What interpersonal skills would you need to facilitate further discussion?
- What concerns do you have and how will you approach these?
- Are there any documents or guidance you would use to aid your clinical decision-making? What are your safeguarding responsibilities?

**How would you support Sarah?**

..........................................................................................................................

..........................................................................................................................

..........................................................................................................................

..........................................................................................................................

..........................................................................................................................

..........................................................................................................................

..........................................................................................................................

..........................................................................................................................

..........................................................................................................................

..........................................................................................................................

..........................................................................................................................

..........................................................................................................................

..........................................................................................................................

..........................................................................................................................

Case Study 2

Derek is a 65-year-old man. He has been married to a woman for 40 years. Derek regularly engages in sex with other men; his family are unaware of this. Derek is attending your clinical area for emergency guidance and advice, as he was raped by a man 2 hours ago. He is very concerned regarding confidentiality.

**How would you support Derek, what advice would you give? What is your responsibility?**

..................................................................................................................

..................................................................................................................

..................................................................................................................

..................................................................................................................

..................................................................................................................

..................................................................................................................

..................................................................................................................

..................................................................................................................

..................................................................................................................

..................................................................................................................

..................................................................................................................

..................................................................................................................

..................................................................................................................

..................................................................................................................

..................................................................................................................

..................................................................................................................

..................................................................................................................

# References

Birchall, J. (2020) Child, Early and Forced Marriage in Fragile and Conflict Affected States. Available at: 805_Child_Early_and_Forced_Marriage_in_FCAS.pdf (ids.ac.uk)

Chen, J., Walters, M. L., Gilbert, L. K. and Patel, N. (2020) 'Sexual violence, stalking, and intimate partner violence by sexual orientation, United States', *Psychology of Violence*, 10(1), pp. 110–119.

Cohen, D. (2017) 'The ties that bind: How armed groups use violence to socialize fighters', *Journal of Peace Research*, 54(5), pp. 701–714.

David, E. J. R. (2014) *Internalised Oppression: The Psychology of Marginalized Groups*. Washington: Springer Publishing Company.

Doncaster Council (2022) Gypsy Roma Traveller Domestic Abuse Worker Application. Available at: https://doncaster.moderngov.co.uk/ieDecisionDetails.aspx?Id=2554

Donnelly, P. (2019) *Wedded to warfare: Forced Marriage in Rebel Groups*. PhD Dissertation. Medford, MA: Tuft University.

Elbert, T., Hinkel, H., Maedl, A., Hermaenau, K. and Hecker, T. (2013) Sexual and Gender-Based Violence in the Kivu Provinces of the Democratic Republic of Congo: Insights from Former Combatants. Available at: https://www.vivo.org/wp-content/uploads/2015/05/LOGiCA_SGBV_DRC_Kivu.pdf

Flanders, C. E., Anderson, A. E. and Tarasoff, L. A. (2020) 'Young bisexual people's experiences of sexual violence: A mixed-methods study', *Journal of Bisexuality*, 20(2), pp. 202–232. https://doi.org/10.1080/15299716.2020.1791300

Flanders, C. E., VanKim, N., Anderson, R. E. and Tarasoff, L. A. (2023) 'Exploring potential determinants of sexual victimization disparities among young sexual minoritized people: A mixed-method Study', *American Psychological Association*, 10(2), pp. 232–245.

Home Office (2023) Female Genital Mutilation Available at: https://www.gov.uk/government/collections/female-genital-mutilation accessed 2nd August 2023

Hughes, T., McCabe, S. E., Wilsnack, S. C., West, B. T. and Boyd, C. J. (2010) 'Victimization and substance use disorders in a national sample of heterosexual and sexual minority women and men', *Addiction*, 105(12), pp. 2130–2140.

Independent Commission for Aid Impact (ICAI) (2020) Literature Review: Conflict-Related Sexual Violence and Sexual Exploitation and Abuse. Available at: https://icai.independent.gov.uk/html-version/psvi-2/

International Committee of The Red Cross (2016) Q&A: Sexual Violence in Armed Conflict. Available at: Q&A: Sexual Violence in Armed Conflict | International Committee of the Red Cross (icrc.org)

James, S. E., Hermann, J. L., Rankin, S., Keisling, M., Mottet, L. and Anafi, M. (2016) The Report of the 2015 U.S. Transgender Survey. National Center for Transgender Equality.

Koos, C. (2017) 'Sexual violence in armed conflicts: Research progress and remaining gaps', *Third World Quarterly*, 38 (9), pp. 1935–1951. https://dx.doi.org/10.1080/01436597.2017.1322461

Maddux, T. and Labrosse, D. (Eds.) (2018) Rape During Civil War. Available at: https://issforum.org/ISSF/PDF/ISSF-Roundtable-10-20.pdf

Mahmood, H. (2016) Child Marriage in Kurdistan Region – Iraq. Available at: UNFPA Iraq | Child Marriage in Kurdistan Region – Iraq

Murad Code (2022) Murad Code Project. Available at: https://www.muradcode.com/#:~:text=%E2%80%A2%20The%20Murad%20Code%3A%20a%20global%20code%20of,place%20survivors%E2%80%99%20rights%20and%20well-being%20at%20its%20heart

Nagel, R. U. (2021) 'Conflict-related sexual violence and the re-escalation of lethal violence', *International Studies Quarterly*, 65, pp. 56–68.

Patten, P. (2022) *War's oldest and least-condemned crime*. Available at: https://news.un.org/en/story/2022/04/1116192

Salter, M. (2012) 'The role of ritual in the organised abuse of children', *Child Abuse Review*, 21, pp. 440–451. https://doi.org/10.1002/car.2215

Schroder, J., Nick, S., Richter-Appelt, H. and Briken, P. (2020) 'Demystifying ritual abuse – Insights by self-identified victims and health care professionals', *Journal of Trauma & Dissociation*, 21(3), pp. 349–364. https://doi.org/10.1080/15299732.2020.1719260

Sevelius, J. M., Gutierrez-Mock, L., Zamudio-Haas, S., McCree, B., Ngo, A., Jackson, A., Clynes, C., Venegas, L., Salinas, A., Herrera, C., Stein, E., Operario, D. and Gamarel, K. (2020) 'Research with marginalized communities: Challenges to continuity during the COVID-19 pandemic', *AIDS Behaviour*, 24(7), pp. 2009–2012. https://doi.org/10.1007/s10461-020-02920-3. PMID: 32415617; PMCID: PMC7228861.

Stachow, E. (2020) 'Conflict-related sexual violence: A review', *British Medical Journal of Military Health*, 166, pp. 183–187. https://doi.org/10.1136/jramc-2019-001376

Swaine, A. (2017) Conflict-Related Sexual Violence in Asia-Pacific. Putting Survivors First. Available at: WPS-00-FINAL-CRSV-PACKAGE.pdf (unwomen.org)

United Kingdom Government (2021) Ensuring the Rights and Wellbeing of Children Born of Sexual Violence in Conflict: Call to Action. Available at: https://www.gov.uk/government/publications/ensuring-the-rights-and-wellbeing-of-children-born-of-sexual-violence-in-conflict-call-to-action

United Kingdom Government (2022) International Ministerial Conference on Preventing Sexual Violence in Conflict Initiative (PSVI) 2022: An Overview. Available at: https://www.gov.uk/government/publications/international-ministerial-conference-on-preventing-sexual-violence-in-conflict-initiative-2022-overview/international-ministerial-conference-on-preventing-sexual-violence-in-conflict-initiative-psvi-2022-an-overview

United Nations (UN) (2022) Conflict-Related Sexual Violence. Available at: https://peacekeeping.un.org/en/conflict-related-sexual-violence

United Nations Office of the Special Representative of the Secretary General on Sexual Violence in Conflict (UNOSRSG) (2022) Framework for the Prevention of Conflict-Related Sexual Violence. Available at: https://reliefweb.int/report/world/framework-prevention-conflict-related-sexual-violence

What Works (2019) Research to Action Toolkit: VAWG in Conflict and Humanitarian Settings. Available at: What Works – Project Resources

Women for Women International (2017) Women for Women International Policy Briefing: Violence Against Women. Available at: wfwi_vaw_policy_briefing_nov_2017.pdf (womenforwomen.org.uk)

World Health Organisation (WHO) (2023) Female Genital Mutilation. Available at: https://www.who.int/news-room/fact-sheets/detail/female-genital-mutilation.

# 8    Supporting Survivors of Sexual Violence and Abuse

The aim of this chapter is to explore how healthcare professionals can practically and emotionally support survivors of sexual violence and abuse (SVA). As has been established throughout this book, SVA is not about sex or a sexual relationship, it is mostly about power, control, humiliation; it can often be influenced by culture, lack of awareness and fear of repercussions of not engaging in certain types of SVA (here, we are talking about cultural circumstance where people are fearful of not engaging in certain practices such as female genital mutilation (FGM) and forced marriage, for example). Experiencing any of these can also be described as experiencing a traumatic event.

## Trauma

Trauma refers to an emotional or psychological response to an event or experience that is deeply distressing or disturbing. Traumatic events are typically characterised by their overwhelming nature, exceeding a person's ability to maintain daily aspects of their life, often leaving them feeling helpless, fearful or powerless. Trauma can result from various types of experiences, including

- Acute trauma: This involves a single traumatic event; it is a specific type of trauma that occurs within a relatively short timeframe, typically involving a sudden and unexpected incident, for example, a natural disaster, a serious accident, physical assault or witnessing violence.
- Chronic trauma: This refers to repeated or prolonged exposure to distressing events, such as ongoing abuse, domestic violence or living in a war zone.
- Complex trauma: This is typically associated with exposure to multiple and interrelated traumatic experiences, often occurring early in life, such as childhood abuse, neglect or growing up in a dysfunctional family environment.

Traumatic experiences can have a profound impact on an individual's mental, emotional and physical well-being. Some common symptoms and reactions to trauma are described as post-traumatic stress (PTS) and can be described as follows:

- Flashbacks or intrusive memories: Reliving the traumatic event through distressing and vivid recollections or nightmares.
- Avoidance behaviours: Trying to avoid reminders of the trauma, which may involve avoiding certain places, people or activities.

DOI: 10.4324/9781003225461-8

- Hyper-arousal: Feeling constantly on edge, being easily startled, having difficulty sleeping or experiencing irritability and anger.
- Emotional numbness: Feeling emotionally detached, having difficulty experiencing positive emotions or experiencing a sense of emptiness.
- Hypervigilance: Being excessively alert and watchful for potential threats or danger.
- Negative self-perception: Feeling guilty, ashamed or blaming oneself for the traumatic event.
- Social withdrawal and isolation: Withdrawing from social activities, feeling disconnected from others or experiencing difficulties in forming and maintaining relationships.

## Trauma Responses

PTS is a normal automated response to being exposed (and re-exposed) to a potentially life-threatening traumatic experience (Ressler et al., 2022). It is a debilitating condition that produces behaviours that can impact behaviour, contribute to hyper-arousal in days, months and years following exposure to trauma. Common PTS indicators can include re-experiencing traumatic memories (flashbacks), avoidance both cognitively and behaviourally of traumatic reminders (such as locations, people, smells etc.), alongside a persistent sense of threat (Villalta et al., 2020). They describe some of the symptoms mentioned above into three categories: (1) emotion dysregulation (for example, heightened emotional reactivity, impulse behaviours, under controlled anger and/or irritability, self-harm), (2) negative self-concept (low self-esteem, feelings of being defeated or worthless) and (3) interpersonal problems (persistent preoccupation or avoidance of social engagement, difficulties in sustaining relationships, lack of productivity at work, self-neglect [physically and emotionally]).

It is recognised that everyone reacts differently to situations and those situations do not have to be life threatening for someone to be affected. The term rape-related PTS (RR-PTS) is also used in the literature when referring to PTS as a result of sexual violence and abuse (SVA); this is a reaction and response to being exposed to any type of sexual violence, as an adult or child. PTS is the term most commonly associated with the effects of experiencing trauma, no matter the trauma; therefore, it could be suggested that putting a 'rape' label on this term does not do anything to differentiate the diagnosis, just highlight the cause, which may deter survivors from accessing healthcare care services due to fear of being judged or reliving the experience. Therefore, identifying as experiencing PTS allows the survivors to demonstrate to the professional; they are experiencing trauma responses without feeling pressured to disclose the sexual violence.

There is no single response to SVA; everyone will respond differently because the circumstance of their assault/experience is different. However, what we do know is that most survivors will display or engage in trauma responses and the severity of PTS in those who have experienced SVA is often higher (Birkeland, Skar and Jensen, 2021). The physiological process is caused when the amygdala (the structure in the temporal lobe thought to process fearful and threatening stimuli) holds on to this emotional reaction attached to the experience and uses it in the future to protect the person from danger when faced with a flashback or something that triggers a reminder of the experience. Whilst a normal response to trauma, it is detrimental to health and well-being. It is therefore important to know that with appropriate psychological support this response can be overturned to ensure traumatic information is processed in a way that creates safety and healing for the survivor; this is aided by a trauma-informed approach to care and practice. Further on in this chapter you will find space to document some national support and local services that may be beneficial in your signposting and supporting of survivors.

PTS can affect approximately 3 in 100 people (National Institute for Health and Care Excellence [NICE], 2022); however, these statistics are significantly increased in those who have experienced SVA with an estimated one in two survivors expected to demonstrate symptoms consistent with PTS. Some address this and seek support. However, most attempt to mask the symptoms using a variety of coping mechanisms such as drugs, alcohol, working excessive hours and more (as mentioned above, Villalta et al., 2020).

## Response to Trauma

The natural response, for most people, to a potentially life-threatening situation is to set off a flight, freeze, fight, flop and friend reaction (Rape Crisis, 2022b). The main function of this is to instinctively keep us safe (survival) and protect us from further harm.

**Fight:** physically fighting, pushing, struggling and fighting verbally, e.g., saying 'no'.
**Flight:** including running, hiding or backing away.
**Freeze:** this is the most common reaction to SVA. Going tense, still and silent is not giving consent.
**Flop:** like freezing, except muscles become loose and the body goes floppy. This is an automatic reaction that can reduce the physical pain of what is happening. The mind can also shut down to protect itself.
**Friend:** calling for a 'friend' or bystander for help, and/or 'befriending' the person who is dangerous, for example, by placating, negotiating, bribing or pleading with them. Again, this is not consent; it is an instinctive response to self-protect.

When faced with these life-threatening experiences or reliving the account of an attack, the physiological process is as follows:

- Adrenaline is released from the adrenal glands; this immediately increases the heart rate.
- Red blood cells are flooded with oxygen and diverted to wherever the body thinks it is needed.
- The lack of oxygen to the brain causes it to only be able to focus on fight or flight.
- Lungs dilate to get more oxygen, causing rapid breathing.
- Sweating takes place to allow the body to cool down following this rapid blood flow causing it to heat up.
- In some: Bowels become looser, vomiting may occur, urinating can become urgent in readiness to make us lighter.
- With the increased heart rate comes increased blood pressure, giving more blood to the muscles in readiness to run or defend themself.

In order to survive, part of the brain holds every detail of the attack in its memory. This mechanism is the main element of what triggers flashbacks and panic attacks. This causes the person to potentially be at risk of experiencing these symptoms every time they are exposed to a signal (emotions or environments) that replicated any element of the attack (for example, a smell, sound or being touched in a certain place/way). It is therefore understandable that to negate these responsive reminders people often engage in the behaviour mentioned above.

As a health care professional(HCP) it is important to know what trauma response is, and how it effects a person, as often these symptoms of trauma response (such as PTS) may be the reason your patient is engaging with your service in the first place. The disclosure often comes later once trust and safety has been built. A better appreciation of the biopsychosocial repercussions of SVA will aid in developing a more holistic and individualised approach to care and support (Chivers-Wilson, 2006).

### Secondary Victimisation/Re-Exposure to Trauma

Secondary victimisation refers to the additional harm or distress experienced by individuals who have already been victimised or traumatised, typically in the context of the legal or criminal justice system. It occurs when victims of crime or abuse encounter insensitive or negative reactions from professionals, institutions or society. These exacerbate their feelings of distrust, abandonment and disappointment following experiences of SVA. It is important to know that survivors of SVA do not need to have reported their experience to the police in order to experience secondary victimisation. In healthcare services we are trained to undertake medical/social history assessments at most appointments, and we see it as essential to explore patients' experiences to get a full indication of the needs they may have. Whilst this is appropriate in most settings, the lack of consistency in accessing HCPs and integrated note keeping can be extremely upsetting to service users; it can be re-triggering and therefore distressing. Re-traumatisation can be described as inadvertently re-creating some conditions or memories of previous trauma that cause an individual to relive the traumatic experience in that moment. Secondary victimisation can result in re-traumatisation.

Secondary victimisation can manifest in various ways, including

- Blaming the survivors: *Survivors may face blame, disbelief or scepticism about their experiences or the severity of the trauma they have endured. This can lead to feelings of guilt, shame or self-doubt and self-blame.*
- Re-traumatisation: *Insensitive questioning or inappropriate handling of survivor's disclosure can cause them to relive the trauma, worsening their psychological and emotional well-being.*
- Lack of support: *Survivors may feel abandoned or unsupported by authorities, healthcare providers or support services. Inadequate access to resources, information or counselling can impede their recovery and perpetuate feelings of isolation and lack of belief.*
- Stigmatisation: *Some survivors may experience social stigma or negative labelling, which can further marginalise and isolate them from their communities.*
- Inadequate legal processes: *Lengthy delays, complex procedures and an absence of clear communication about the progress of legal cases can contribute to survivors' feelings of frustration, powerlessness and a lack of closure.*

Re-victimisation can also refer to the risk or experience of future assaults (Walsh, 2012). Some studies have identified that women who have been raped are seven times more likely to be raped again, compared to those who have never experienced SVA (Acierno et al., 1999).

Addressing secondary victimisation requires the implementation of a victim-centred trauma-informed approach, as well as public awareness and education initiatives to foster understanding of the impact of SVA. Efforts from HCPs should focus on empowering survivors, providing appropriate support services and improving the sensitivity and responsiveness of all involved in their care.

## Trauma-Informed Approaches

It is clear, from the limited literature we have explored throughout this book so far, that there is a need for HCPs to be more informed about trauma when it comes to supporting SVA, both pre- and post-disclosure. Quadara (2015) suggests that being in the moment to fully support survivors can only be undertaken by HCPs being trauma-informed within their care and in their practice. We have already highlighted that the effects of being exposed to distressing or harmful circumstances or events result in trauma; therefore, trauma is the effect rather than the event (Isobel, 2016). For survivors of SVA, the absence of HCPs being trained in trauma-informed approaches (TiA) often results in fragmented services and re-traumatisation (Dworkin and Schumacher, 2016). Being trauma-informed puts the full focus towards the experience and needs of the survivor. In fact, research increasingly is suggesting that all HCPs need to be providing trauma-informed care (TiC) and practice (TiCP) to make any impact on improving all health outcomes, specifically surrounding public health implications (The Kings Fund, 2019). Sweeney and Taggart (2018) state that whilst there is international interest, TiA can be complex to embed in services, with a lack of understanding often causing most services to suggest they are already trauma-informed when they are not. Trauma-informed approaches can potentially lead to a fundamental shift on how services are organised and delivered, a thread that has been supported by the NHS Long Term Plan (2019) but does not seem to have grown in trajectory. In November 2022 the UK Office for Health Improvement and Disparities provided clarity of a working definition of trauma-informed practice. This framework established the key principles and integration of TiA in the health and social care sector.

Trauma-informed approaches have a range of literature noting of its benefit, and this evidence base is growing exponentially. The police in the UK are being educated at their basic entry level of training to be trauma-informed and the Department for Levelling Up, Housing and Communities have also produced a framework to include TiA to support people experiencing multiple disadvantages. The integration of TiA solidifies the awareness trauma had on an individual's life. This is mainly because of the amount of contact public health authorities have with people who have mental health issues. It could be argued, however, that the majority of patients that HCPs come into contact with also have mental health issues; nearly all will have experienced trauma to some degree and that trauma experience will be a contributing factor to their poor mental health. This therefore suggests that there should be consistency in our approaches to education for first responders and public service providers. TIA should be embedded into healthcare professional education.

## What Is Trauma-Informed Care and Practice

TiCP is a trauma-informed approach originating from the development of research that identified the more adverse events people are exposed to, the greater negative impact they will have on all health outcomes. Its approach is underpinned by strengths-based principles and grounded in an understanding of the impact trauma has on the individual. It involves creating opportunities for people to become empowered to rebuild their sense of personal control (Hopper, Bassuk, and Olivet, 2010). The key principles of trauma-informed approaches are defined by the Centre for Disease Control and Prevention (2020) as follows:

1 Safety
2 Trustworthiness and transparency
3 Peer support
4 Collaboration and mutuality
5 Empowerment and choice
6 Cultural, historical and gender issues

These principles are reflected in the UK government's identification of their six principles, as outlined in Table 8.1:.

*Table 8.1* Principles of Trauma-Informed Approaches

| | |
|---|---|
| Safety | The physical, psychological and emotional safety of service users and staff is prioritised, by <br><br> • people knowing they are safe or asking what they need to feel safe <br> • there being reasonable freedom from threat or harm <br> • attempting to prevent re-traumatisation <br> • putting policies, practices and safeguarding arrangements in place |
| Trustworthiness | Transparency exists in an organisation's policies and procedures, with the objective of building trust among staff, service users and the wider community, by <br><br> • the organisation and staff explaining what they are doing and why <br> • the organisation and staff doing what they say they will do <br> • expectations being made clear and the organisation and staff not overpromising |
| Choice | Service users are supported in shared decision-making, choice and goal setting to determine the plan of action they need to heal and move forward, by <br><br> • ensuring service users and staff have a voice in the decision-making process of the organisation and its services <br> • listening to the needs and wishes of service users and staff <br> • explaining choices clearly and transparently <br> • acknowledging that people who have experienced or are experiencing trauma may feel a lack of safety or control over the course of their life which can cause difficulties in developing trusting relationships |
| Collaboration | The value of staff and service user experience is recognised in overcoming challenges and improving the system as a whole, by <br><br> • using formal and informal peer support and mutual self-help <br> • the organisation asking service users and staff what they need and collaboratively considering how these needs can be met <br> • focusing on working alongside and actively involving service users in the delivery of services |

*(Continued)*

*Table 8.1* (Continued)

| | |
|---|---|
| Empowerment | Efforts are made to share power and give service users and staff a strong voice in decision-making, at both individual and organisational levels, by<br><br>• validating feelings and concerns of staff and service users<br>• listening to what a person wants and needs<br>• supporting people to make decisions and take action<br>• acknowledging that people who have experienced or are experiencing trauma may feel powerless to control what happens to them, isolated by their experiences and have feelings of low self-worth |
| Cultural considerations | Move past cultural stereotypes and biases based on, for example, gender, sexual orientation, age, religion, disability, geography, race or ethnicity by<br><br>• offering access to gender-responsive services<br>• leveraging the healing value of traditional cultural connections<br>• incorporating policies, protocols and processes that are responsive to the needs of individuals served |

*Source*: Gov.UK (2022).

Many mental and physical illnesses, and general emotional distress are now thought to be associated with unprocessed traumatic experiences (Felitti and Anda, 1997; Anda et al., 2010; Nelson, 2020). The goal of TiC is also to avoid re-traumatising someone (Quadara, 2015) through re-exposure to trauma. It is apparent that HCPs are inadvertently subjecting survivors to relive their trauma at different stages of the disclosure, as they navigate through health areas. The benefits of a trauma-informed workforce are significant when considering the implications of poor support, both in terms of the survivors' health and well-being, and the cost to the NHS.

The NHS (2018) published a 'radial' strategic direction for sexual assault and abuse services with an aim of lifelong care for victims and survivors. This document emphasised the importance of having a trauma-informed workforce. Unfortunately, the focus of their strategic aims is on specialist services, such as those who carry out medical and forensic examinations and provide specialist practical and emotional support (counselling, psychology and voluntary organisations that provide emotional support) services. However, this document demonstrates a lack of insight into the needs of the 'general' healthcare workforce when it comes to supporting survivors of SVA. Therefore, this 'radical' strategic document fails to recognise that, whilst the services they identify are exceptionally important in providing specialist care, general and frontline HCPs that work outside of these environments are essentially key to providing immediate support to survivors (both following disclosure and in addressing any impacts of PTS that the person may be seeking support for) and will go on to encourage signposting and engagement in those specialist areas. This demonstrates a big disconnect in who the policy leaders are aiming their approaches and resources towards. As such, this lack of insight has implication for both survivors and HCPs.

### How You can Engage in and Implement Trauma-Informed Approached in Your Practice

Individual practitioners can implement TiCP, even when they do not work in trauma-informed organisations (Sweeney et al., 2019) however, research indicates that to undertake this approach in the most appropriate way, change is required at a cultural and strategic level, not just an organisational one (Sweeney et al., 2016; Harris and Fallot, 2001). Despite the requirement to embed asking about experiences of trauma and abuse, reported rates of asking are low (Xiao et al., 2016); this was reflected in the discussions in Chapter 3, with research indicating practitioners often do not screen for SVA experiences. It may be that HCPs struggle to talk about trauma in general, rather than just SVA, and worry that asking about difficult, distressing and dangerous events may overwhelm both themselves and service users. This area of practice needs further research to fully explore the barriers. Only then can we provide the correct education and training to ensure practitioners are well prepared to support disclosures of SVA. In the meantime, as a practitioner there are numerous ways you can explore embedding TiCP in your clinical environment to improve experience for survivors. Below are a few ideas on how to do so:

- Educate yourself to enhance your understanding of TiCP.
- Enquire with your clinical leads or education leads to see if your organisation is adopting TiCP into their clinical approaches, if so, where? Explore how they are doing this and whether it can be replicated.
- Using your CPD hours, are there any internal or external teaching sessions/masterclasses, modules specifically focusing on TiCP you could access?
- It is important that you understand the theoretical underpinning of these approaches; however, start embedding them into your practice after reading this book. Consider your language and assessment questions you use with your service users, how could they be re-directed in a more trauma-informed way.
- This is a difficult point, but an important one, have you experienced SVA? Does it impact how you would ask about trauma? Are you worried that opening this line of conversation may be triggering for you? If so, you might want to find support for your needs via your general practitioner, occupational support or a voluntary organisation such as rape crisis.

### Sexual Assault Referral Centres

If someone has experienced SVA, there must be a consideration of whether forensic evidence needs to be looked for. In the aftermath of SVA, all people regardless of age or gender should have access to a timely forensic examination. For some this will be a choice, and therefore, a discussion you will need to facilitate. However, for others (cases of child sex abuse and those that lack capacity), a specialist service will have those discussions. To explore this, you must have an awareness of where (in your region) those specialist services are; your organisation's safeguarding lead will be able to help you compile a list of services. You can also find your nearest SARC in the NHS website at the following link: https://www.nhs.uk/service-search/other-services/Rape-and-sexual-assault-referral-centres/LocationSearch/364

Sexual assault referral centres offer medical, emotional and practical support to anyone who has been raped or sexually abused by specially trained nurses and/or medical staff, within a particular timeframe. They are specifically designed to ensure the survivor is as comfortable as they can be, and staff are fully educated to ensure they can help the survivor make an informed decision about what they want to do next. Most SARCs will also have specially trained Independence Sexual Violence Advisors (ISVA) who provide a range of specialist support which will follow through a survivor's legal proceedings, should they wish to report their assault to the police.

## Forensic Intervention

The aim of a high-quality forensic intervention will be to

- address the survivors' concerns (including STI and pregnancy risk – usually signposting to a sexual health centre)
- collection of evidence
- minimise trauma
- aid and support recovery

Some survivors of SVA may be unable to make an immediate decision about whether they wish to report the assault. Engaging in SARC and forensic examinations provides both the police and the survivor with the best possible opportunity to recover evidence for use within a criminal investigation, if the person so chooses, and minimises the risk of a miscarriage of justice such as

a   the risk of wrongful conviction(s);
b   wrongful acquittal(s); or
c   obstructing or delaying investigation(s).

However, the pressure to report can also cause barriers to engagement in these services. Therefore, it should be made clear that should your service user refer themself (alone or via you) to a SARC, they can change their mind following the initial discussion about what to expect or what their choices are. They can also have the forensic examination undertaken and then decide to report their assault to the police later; many SARCs can store evidence from examinations for certain periods of time, or until the survivor wishes to report the assault to the police. It should also be noted at this point that referral to a SARC and reporting to the police do not come hand in hand. The SARC is there to support and facilitate police referral but not inform them regardless (unless there is a safeguarding risk and/or the survivor is a child).

Most frequently, examinations are undertaken in a SARC or specialist SVA unit; however, they may also be carried out within local NHS or police (patient examination suits) premises.

## Timescales for Medical and Forensic Care

### *Emergency Medical Needs Always Outweigh the Need to Collect Evidence*

If someone has injuries from their assault that indicates the need for immediate treatment, this must be prioritised above evidence collection. This will be noted as part of the forensic collection process with regard to highlighting some risk for cross contamination. Clothing, tampons, toothbrushes etc. can all be saved to provide evidence, and if you see a survivor immediately after their experience, it is important to remember this (for example, do not give them a drink of water if they are considering forensic examination as oral evidence may need to be taken). Evidence bags would be used to collect items and chain of evidence must be adhered to; this is not always practical in some healthcare environments, which is why it is often best to suggest SARC referral initially, until the survivor has decided whether they would like to report their experience. Table 8.2 provides an overview of the medical considerations that must be addressed:

*Table 8.2* Medical Considerations Following Sexual Violence and Abuse

| Care | Timescale | Where to Get This |
| --- | --- | --- |
| Forensic medical examination | Forensic window period<br>Vaginal penetration 10 days<br>Anal penetration 72 hours<br>Oral penetration 48 hours<br>Digital (i.e., finger) penetration 48 hours<br>*please note this may differ across regions/countries. Always get advice from your local SARC for their timescales* | Sexual assault referral centres |
| HIV risk assessment<br>Post-exposure prophylaxis (PEP) is a combination of HIV drugs that can prevent the virus taking hold | HIV risk assessment should be conducted within 72 hours of assault and consideration given to HIV PEP. PEP is only given to people who meet the guidelines and must be taken within 72 hours of exposure to the virus to be effective | This risk assessment can be carried out at a SARC, sexual health service and emergency departments (at weekends and evenings if there is no sexual health access) |
| Pregnancy risk | Emergency contraception is available until **five days** post-assault and can include consideration for an intrauterine contraceptive device (IUD) such as a copper coil – timescale for IUD is dependent on where the individual is in their cycle and if there is any previous pregnancy risk | Most SARCs can offer emergency contraception, and survivors may have to attend a sexual health clinic or their GP for an IUD |

## Aftercare

Screening for sexually transmitted infections (STI) is often undertaken at either sexual health clinics or primary caregivers (i.e., GP practices). Whilst some forensic examinations can include STI screening, it is often not part of the procedure due to incubation period for most infections and the impact STI screening may have on cases that go to court.

## Safeguarding Adults, Young People and Children

Safeguarding in cases of SVA can be incredibly complex. Whether to involve or refer to safeguarding teams is a decision you may need to make either during or following supporting a survivor of SVA. This book is focused on supporting survivors of SVA, and whilst that does need to acknowledge the safeguarding implications, it is essential to be aware of the legal parameters of types of SVA and national guidelines in your country, alongside your own organisations' safeguarding team roles and responsibilities. Ensure your safeguarding mandatory training linked to your organisation is up to date as this will aid in providing you with the most contemporary guidance. For essential further reading, please see Keeling and Goosy's (2021) *Safeguarding Across the Life Span*, an excellent resource for HCPs.

In the context of healthcare, safeguarding is a relatively new phenomenon. Whilst protecting the 'vulnerable' has always been in the mindset of healthcare, it was not always in a healthy way, for example, the 'poor' being sent to workhouses to protect them from indolence and starvation, the confinement of single mothers to institutions for displaying symptoms of what we now know is post-natal depression, or simply to 'protect their chastity' further. Safeguarding in the current context (specifically in the UK) took on a new meaning within the realms of professional responsibility following both the introduction of the Mental Health Act (1982) and the Children Act (1989).

Safeguarding is an interdisciplinary and interprofessional process. Co-operation, communication and information sharing between professionals and agencies are essential for improved outcomes.

If you have any concerns regarding safeguarding with your service users in a healthcare setting, there are a number of avenues, you can seek advice and support from

- Most departments in healthcare organisations will have departmental designated safeguarding leads. This is usually a member of staff who has additional responsibilities to support others when they are in need of advice, and to keep their department policies' folders/staff up to date with any changes to policies etc.
- The organisation you work for will (usually) also have a designated safeguarding team. You can contact this team for advice if you are not sure if there are safeguarding needs, or to report safeguarding concerns.
- All local authorities also have designated safeguarding teams; here you can report suspected abuse as a practitioner and/or a member of the public. They're often referred to as Safeguarding Adult Board/Safeguarding Children Partnerships.
- NHS safeguarding app: The NHS safeguarding app has been developed to act as a comprehensive resource for healthcare professionals, carers and citizens. It provides 24-hour, mobile access on up-to-date legislation and guidance across the safeguarding life course. It can be accessed via Apple iOS or Google Play or by searching 'NHS Safeguarding'.
- If you feel anyone is in immediate danger, call the emergency services (in the UK this is 999).

## Legal Parameters

The authors of this book work primarily across England; therefore, the legal parameters explored are in relation to English law. It is important you are aware of country differences.

Incidences where you legally have a responsibility to report SVA to the relevant authorities in England are outlined in Table 8.3:

## Communication

If someone presents in the healthcare system and discloses SVA, it is important that this is taken seriously, and in line with the correct system policies and protocols. However, many places do not have specific policies, especially around adult disclosures of SVA. Therefore, gathering information is essential to determine how you may support the individual. It is important that time is taken by the HCP to listen to the person's disclosure and respond with the appropriate tone and information. The following key skills will aid in your communication.

*Table 8.3* Legal Responsibilities in Reporting Disclosures of Sexual Violence and Abuse

| SVA | Agency/Organisation | Other People You (or Your Safeguarding Lead) Must Communicate With |
| --- | --- | --- |
| SVA in children 17 or under | • Local authority safeguarding board | • Your organisations' safeguarding team<br>• Police |
| Female genital mutilation (under 18s) | • Police | • Your organisations' safeguarding team<br>• Local authority safeguarding boards |
| Forced marriage | • Your organisations' safeguarding team | • Forced Marriage Unit fmu@fcdo.gov.uk<br>• Police<br>• Local authority safeguarding boards |
| Adults 'at risk' or/and lack capacity | • Your organisations' safeguarding team | • Local authority safeguarding boards<br>• Police |

### Active Listening

Active listening is the process of listening to someone with your full attention, using all your senses with the aim of understating the person in front of you. This means considering your position (try to remove physical barriers), your facial expressions, the tone of your voice and ignoring other distractions (external factors). It is acceptable to tell the survivors that you appreciate they have shared their experience; however, this consultation may take longer than expected so you are going to tell your colleagues to not disturb you/or to re-allocate your next patient, if possible. Then you can return and give that person your full attention. Otherwise, they will pick up on your distractions and it may prevent them from disclosing further or accepting support as often distraction manifest as lack of belief or lack of importance applied to their experience (Dosdale, 2023).

Active listening is aligned with TiCP and involves trying to understand what is going on for them and what they want to communicate to you. It's about getting alongside someone's concerns and being  Some principles of active listening are outlined below:

- Any questions should be open v' closed.
- Reflect on what they have said, paraphrase it back and clarify/summarise to ensure understanding and demonstrate you have been listening.
- Minimal encouragers, let them talk.
- Use positive body language: nod, eye contact.
- Show empathy.

The following barriers to active listening are worth considering:

- lack of interest
- partial listening due to distraction
- pre-judgemental thoughts
- previous experience of SVA (if this impacts your ability to be an active lister to survivors of SVA, consider referring to another colleague
- lack of understanding of cultural differences
- unconscious bias
- stereotypical reaction (excessive anger or shock)/overreactive
- sharing your experiences of SVA

Main aspects to remember when supporting survivors of SVA are as follows:

**Do:**

- Stay calm.
- Express empathy.
- Explore whether they are in immediate danger.
- Allow them to stay in control of what they are disclosing.
- Guide to support and ask them what they would like to happen next.
- Be open and transparent if you have safeguarding concerns.
- Ask what support they have at home/with friends and/or family.

**Don't:**

- Overreact or show excessive shock and/or anger.
- Do not minimise the experience.
- Do not blame the individual in any way or doubt their experience, that is not part of your role.
- You do not need to take control or make unrealistic promises.
- Do not ask for more details or specific information about the assault if it is not needed.

**Self-Completion Section**

*Organisations that Will Support Survivors*

Below is space that aims at providing a resource for you to explore and document organisations that you may use to signpost your survivors to.

---

**National organisations:**

..............................................................................................................................

..............................................................................................................................

..............................................................................................................................

..............................................................................................................................

..............................................................................................................................

..............................................................................................................................

..............................................................................................................................

..............................................................................................................................

..............................................................................................................................

..............................................................................................................................

**Regional organisations:**

..........................................................................................................................................

..........................................................................................................................................

..........................................................................................................................................

..........................................................................................................................................

..........................................................................................................................................

..........................................................................................................................................

..........................................................................................................................................

..........................................................................................................................................

..........................................................................................................................................

..........................................................................................................................................

..........................................................................................................................................

## References

Acierno, R., Resnick, H., Kilpatrick, D. G., Saunders, B. and Best, C. L. (1999) 'Risk factors for rape, physical assault, and posttraumatic stress disorder in women: Examination of differential multivariate relationships', *Journal of Anxiety Disorders*, 13(6), pp. 541–563.

Anda, R. F., Butchart, A., Felitti, V. J. and Brown, D. W. (2010) 'Building a framework for global surveillance of the public health implications of adverse childhood experiences', *American Journal of Preventative Medicine*, 39(1), pp. 93–98. https://doi.org/10.1016/j.amepre.2010.03.015

Birkeland, M. S., Skar, A. M. S. and Jensen, T. K. (2021) 'Do different traumatic events invoke different kinds of post-traumatic stress symptoms?', *European Journal of Psychotraumatology*, 12(sup1)

Centre for Disease Control and Prevention (2020) Guiding principles to a trauma-informed approach. Available at: https://www.cdc.gov/orr/infographics/6_principles_trauma_info.htm

Chivers-Wilson, K. A. (2006) 'Sexual assault and posttraumatic stress disorder: A review of the biological, psychological and sociological factors and treatments', *McGill Journal of Medicine*, 9(2), pp. 111–118.

Dosdale, C. (2023) *Adult Experiences of Rape Disclosures in Nursing Practice: A Phenomenological Study*. PhD Thesis. Northumbria University. Available at: https://nrl.northumbria.ac.uk/id/eprint/51579/

Dworkin, E. R. and Schumacher, J. A. (2016) Preventing posttraumatic stress related to sexual assault through early intervention: A systematic review. *Trauma, Violence & Abuse*, 19(4). https://doi.org/10.1177/1524838016669518

Felitti, V. J. and Anda, R. F. (1997) The Adverse Childhood Experiences (ACE) Study. *Centre for Disease Control and Prevention*. Retrieved from http://www.cdc.gov/ace/index.htm

Gov. UK (2019) *The NHS Long Term Plan*. Available online at: https://www.gov.uk/government/news/nhs-long-term-plan-launched (Accessed 24/07/2023)

Gov.UK (2022) *Working definition of Trauma Informed Practice (UK)*. Available at: https://www.gov.uk/government/publications/working-definition-of-trauma-informed-practice/working-definition-of-trauma-informed-practice#:~:text=There%20are%206%20principles%20of,collaboration%2C%20empowerment%20and%20cultural%20consideration

Harris, M. and Fallot, R. D. (2001) *Using Trauma Theory to Design Service Systems*. Farnham, Jossey-Bass/Wiley.

Hopper, E. K., Bassuk, E. L. and Olivet, J. (2010) 'Shelter from the storm: Trauma-informed care in homelessness services settings.', *The Open Health Services and Policy Journal*, 3, pp 80–100.

Isobel, S. (2016), 'Trauma informed care: A radical shift or basic good practice?', *Australasian Psychiatry*, 24(6), pp. 589–591.

Keeling, J. and Goosy, D. (2021) *Safeguarding Across the Life Span*. London, SAGE Publications Ltd.

Kings Fund (2019) *Tackling Poor Health Outcomes: The Role of Trauma-Informed Care*. Available at: https://www.kingsfund.org.uk/blog/2019/11/trauma-informed-care

National Institute for Health and Care Excellence (NICE). (2022) *Post-Traumatic Stress Ddisorder: How Common Is It?* Available online at: https://cks.nice.org.uk/topics/post-traumatic-stress-disorder/background-information/prevalence/

Nelson, C. (2020) 'Adversity in childhood is linked to mental and physical health throughout life', *British Medical Journal*, 371 https://doi.org/10.1136/bmj.m3048

NHS (2018) 'Strategic Direction for Sexual Assault and Abuse Services Lifelong care for victims and survivors: 2018 – 2023' NHS England. Available at: https://www.england.nhs.uk/wp-content/uploads/2018/04/strategic-direction-sexual-assault-and-abuse-services.pdf.

Quadara, A. (2015) *Conceptualising the Prevention of Child Sexual Abuse. Australian Institute of Family Studies*. Available online at: https://aifs.gov.au/research/research-reports/conceptualising-prevention-child-sexual-abuse

Rape Crisis (2022b) *Myths Vs Facts*. Available at: https://rapecrisis.org.uk/get-informed/about-sexual-violence/myths-vs-realities/

Ressler, K. J., Berretta, S., Bolshakov, V. Y., Rosso, I. M., Meloni, E. G., Rauch, S. L. and Carlezon, W. A. Jr (2022) 'Post-traumatic stress disorder: Clinical and translational neuroscience from cells to circuits', *Nature Reviews Neurology*, 18, pp. 273–288.

Sweeney, A., Clement, S., Fitson, B. and Kennedy, A. (2016) Trauma-informed mental healthcare in the UK: what is it and how can we further its development? *Mental Health Review Journal*, 21(3), pp. 174–192. DOI: 10.1108/MHRJ-01-2015-0006

Sweeney, A., Perot, C., Callard, F., Adenden, V., Mantovani, N. and Goldsmith, L. (2019) 'Out of the silence: Towards grassroots and trauma-informed support for people who have experienced sexual violence and abuse', *Epidemiology and Psychiatric Sciences*, 28(6), pp. 598–602.

Sweeney, A. and Taggart, D. (2018) '(Mis)understanding trauma-informed approaches in mental health', *Journal of Mental Health*, 27(5), pp. 383–387.

Villalta, L., Khadr, S., Chua, K. C., Kramer, T., Clarke, V., Viner, R. M., Stringaris, A. and Smith, P. (2020) 'Complex post-traumatic stress symptoms in female adolescents: The role of emotion dysregulation in impairment and trauma exposure after an acute sexual assault', *European Journal of Psychotraumatology*, 11(1), p. 1710400.

Walsh, F. (2012) "Family Resilience: Strengths Forged Through Adversity". In F. Walsh (Ed.), *Normal Family Processes: Growing Diversity and Complexity* (pp. 399–427). Washington, The Guilford Press.

Xiao, C., Gavrilidis, E., Lee, S. and Kulkarni, J. (2016) 'Do mental health clinicians elicit a history of previous trauma in female psychiatric inpatients?', *Journal of Mental Health*, 25, pp. 359–365.

# 9    Practitioner Guidance in Supporting Survivors of Sexual Violence and Abuse

## Introduction

The purpose of this chapter is to consider the impact on practitioners working in roles where they are involved in the identification of sexual violence and abuse (SVA) and in supporting those who are or have experienced it. It is difficult to obtain specific data relating only to health, and therefore, it is necessary to consider this in the wider context of the health and social care workforce.

Healthcare practitioners (HCPs) who witness the heightened emotions of survivors of SVA often suppress their own emotions to remain professional and maintain the therapeutic relationship, with the ability to compartmentalise being considered an essential skill (Dosdale, 2023). It is this skill that Williston and Lafreniere (2013) state helps practitioners to remove the subjectivity from disclosures of intimate personal violence and one that ultimately allows them to engage with their patient, regardless of the outcome of the consultation. However, whilst Dosdale's (2023) study focused only on nurses, an important finding shows that where nurses suppress their own emotions, this impacts negatively their ability to act as an advocate for the survivor, which is a fundamental part of an HCP's role. Further to this, Dosdale (2023) suggests that suppression of emotion can later manifest when professionals reflect back on their experiences and that this can produce a negative impact on the long-term well-being of HCPs. Consequently, HCPs working with those who have experienced SVA must delicately balance their own emotions, alongside those of their patients whilst acting in their best interests.

## Definitions and Terminology

There are many terms used to describe the negative consequences on the well-being of staff who work in challenging roles supporting those who have experienced traumatic events. Recent reviews of the health workforce (Kinman and Teoh, 2018; Kinman, Teoh and Harris, 2020; The Kings Fund 2020) focused on key professional groups (doctors, nurses and midwives) working in the sector and found that there were much higher rates of self-reported mental health problems among these groups than in the general working population. Key concerns about well-being referred to psychological distress, burnout, compassion fatigue, post-traumatic stress (PTS), and increased risk of suicide. Some of the reported impacts of work-related health problems included difficulties sleeping, poor mental health and reduced cognitive function, all of which contribute to potential patient safety impacts.

In order to support HCPs in their support of survivors of SVA, it is important to understand some of the terms used to describe the impacts it has on practitioners:

DOI: 10.4324/9781003225461-9

# Burnout

There is recognition of the experience of burnout among many frontline staff. Burnout is a work-related stress syndrome, and the key features are emotional and physical exhaustion (Wei et al., 2022). Other symptoms include depersonalisation and reduced personal accomplishment. Burnout is cumulative, developing over time, and is linked to the work environment, including shift work, lack of resources and the organisational context, which includes workplace culture. Burnout is mainly attributed to prolonged and excessive stress and, importantly, chronic stress that has not been successfully managed (Health and Social Care Committee, 2021).

Burnout can impact significantly on mental health and can lead to depression and anxiety, substance abuse and increased risk of suicide (Wei et al., 2022). Burnout often results in job dissatisfaction and is cited as a key reason for staff absence as well as for intending to leave their job role (Kinman, 2021). Given the association between burnout and increased risk of professional errors and reduced quality of care delivery, when HCPs continue to work whilst experiencing burnout, there are increased risks to service users. According to Kinman (2021), younger staff are more vulnerable to burnout.

In recent years, the global pandemic has highlighted the pressures faced by the general health and social care workforce, particularly those staff who work in frontline roles. Whilst the pressures have been exacerbated by the pandemic, it is accepted that many of the challenges are not new and there is increasing recognition of the stressful, demanding and often emotional nature of working in these environments.

Prior to the pandemic, a study by McKinley, McCain and Convie (2020) found that a third of the doctors they surveyed described themselves as burned out, and this is the same for many front-line professionals. It is known that work-related stress, anxiety and depression are much more prevalent among those working in the health and social care sector and that rates have been rising steadily since 2016 (Kinman, 2021). Concerns around HCP incidences of suicide and suicide risk have been rising both during and following the COVID-19 pandemic and are deeply concerning (Ross, 2020; Trivedi, 2023). These risks are attributed to many things such as COVID-19, increased work pressures and impact on mental health during this time and following it, cost of living crisis etc. Currently, workforce burnout is described by many as the highest in the history of the NHS and care systems, and as such, it is an extraordinarily dangerous risk to the future functioning of services, individuals and patient safety (Health and Social Care Committee, 2021).

# Impact of Burnout on Healthcare Staff

Whilst it is accepted that not all those working with individuals who have experienced or are at risk of SVA are employed by the NHS, it is difficult to access data about the impact of such work on health and well-being from organisations outside of health and social care. The NHS Staff Survey has been conducted annually since 2003 and is one of the largest workforce surveys in the world. There is no comparable data for those working in the social care sector, but the House of Commons Committees has asked the UK Government to extend the NHS Survey to cover the care sector (House of Commons Committees, 2021). Whilst there is an absence of data in the care sector, the Health and Social Care Committee (2021) outlines that burnout has been raised as a serious problem by many organisations across the care sector. These organisations include those that represent orthopaedic surgeons, dentists, pharmacists, nurses, cardiothoracic surgeons,

Table 9.1 NHS Staff Survey Data in Relation to Burnout

| Workload and Resources | |
| --- | --- |
| 43.2% are able to meet all the conflicting demands on their time | This has declined over 4% and is now at a five-year low (2017: 44.4%, 2018: 44.9%, 2019: 46.1%, 2020: 47.7%) |
| 27.2% said there are enough staff for them to do their job properly | This has declined by over 11% since 2020 |
| 23.5% say they have unrealistic time pressures | |
| 57.3% say they have adequate materials, supplies and equipment to do their work | This is down by 3% since 2020 |
| 57% say their organisation takes positive action on health and well-being | |
| 46.8% of staff have felt unwell as a result of work-related stress in the last 12 months | |
| 34.3% feel burnt out because of their work | This varies across staff groups: Ambulance 51%; Nurses and Midwives 40.5%; Nursing and Healthcare Assistants 38%; Medical and Dental 33.1%; Wider Healthcare Team 25.1% |

anaesthetists, midwives, health visitors and general practitioners, palliative care workers and paediatric intensive care workers, in addition to those representing staff in adult social care.

The NHS Staff Survey (2021) focuses on the experiences of staff working in their respective NHS organisations and includes questions about teamwork and having a voice in the organisation as well as health, well-being and safety of staff. The most recent results from the NHS Staff Survey (2021) were completed by 648,594 staff. Some key data from the survey is presented in Table 9.1.

The NHS Staff Survey (2021) suggests that an unacceptably high number of staff are experiencing negative impacts on health and well-being as a result of stress in the workplace and that the upward trend is worrying. It is accepted that the COVID-19 pandemic has impacted the data captured in the survey. Indeed nine out of ten NHS trust leaders reported being concerned about staff well-being, stress and burnout following the pandemic. However, the survey does provide details of trends, which includes pre-pandemic data, and it is noted that burnout and poor mental well-being of staff in the health sector is both a historic and an ongoing concern.

## Compassion Fatigue

Compassion fatigue was first outlined by Joinson (1992) and relates to HCPs' diminished ability to care, empathise or feel compassion for others because of prolonged and repeated experience of caring for those who are or who have suffered. Whilst this implies compassion fatigue is the result of experiencing many events, it can also arise from the experience of caring for one individual person or from one event (Cavanagh, Cockett and Doig, 2019).

Compassion fatigue is related to vicarious trauma and secondary traumatic stress which both result from exposure to the trauma experienced by others as opposed to experiencing the trauma itself (Cavanagh, Cockett and Doig, 2019). Whilst compassion fatigue and burnout are often used interchangeably, they are distinct. As outlined above, burnout often emerges gradually over time and is linked to work-related attributes, such as excessive workload, whereas compassion fatigue is thought to develop more quickly and is a direct consequence of exposure to traumatic material and the adverse experiences of others. It is therefore considered that whilst anyone in employment can experience burnout as a result of prolonged workplace stressors, and indeed, burnout can contribute to compassion fatigue, compassion fatigue is unique to those involved in caring or providing emotional support to others and is triggered by the need to use empathy and emotional energy.

## Secondary Traumatic Stress

PTS is a mental health condition caused by a traumatic experience. The symptoms of PTS include flashbacks, nightmares, difficulty sleeping as well as feelings of anxiety (Kinman, 2021). Secondary traumatic stress is a stress response that is produced as a consequence of either witnessing or knowing about the trauma experienced by others (Nimmo and Huggard, 2013). It is acknowledged that due to the statistics surrounding SVA, many HCPs will have personally experienced SVA; therefore, there is a need to be mindful of the impact a disclosure may have on your own experiences of trauma and your recovery.

## Vicarious Trauma

Vicarious trauma refers to the undesirable outcomes of working directly with traumatised populations. It is produced in situations where staff engage with service users who have experienced distress and traumatic events; it is a result of listening to and observing the effects of trauma from those who have experienced it, as well as via reviewing case files and evidence and being involved in responding to these experiences (Office for Victims of Crime, 2022). It is often described as a stressful traumatic state that can involve a preoccupation with knowing about the trauma experienced by others.

As outlined so far in this chapter, there are many terms, often used interchangeably and with similarities between them, to describe some of the negative consequences of caring for those who have experienced SVA/trauma. What is clear is that these may be experienced by anyone working in a helping and caring role and that they may result in long-term effects that include impaired ability to perform in the role, as well as to deliver safe and effective care.

## Impact on Empathy

All of the above affect an individual's ability to empathise. Empathy is often described as the ability to understand other people's feelings, and in relation to healthcare, this has many dimensions. Conceptually, empathy is difficult to define from literature as often the terms empathy, compassion and sympathy are used and defined interchangeably. This is because the literature surrounding empathy in healthcare is often referred to in a generic way, as a skill or attribute. Due to empathy being seen as an essential HCP skill and difficult to understand from a clinical perspective, many professionals draw upon personal experiences of what empathy is to influence their skill clinically, for example, HCPs' experience following disclosures of SVA is very much based on their own personal feeling of SVA from a societal perspective (horrid, awful, anger). Empathy within clinical practice tends to be separated into cognitive or emotional empathy (Santo et al., 2014). Cognitive empathy can be defined as taking the perspective of another person. In contrast, emotional empathy is often described as taking on the emotional experiences or feelings of another person. Fernandez and Zahavi (2021) suggest that both concepts can be trained in HCPs. However, much of the literature indicates that emotional empathy is more intuitive and indicative of the role of most HCPs (Hochchild, 2003). The main concern of this discussion is that by producing an understanding and sharing another's feelings/experiences, HCPs can become easily overwhelmed, and it is this type of empathy that is often associated with burnout, distress and compassion fatigue (Duarte, Pinto-Gouveia and Cruz, 2016; Moudatsou et al., 2020; Fernandez and Zahavi, 2021).

Santo et al. (2014) found that when HCPs successfully manage their emotions following interactions with survivors that trigger empathy, they are more satisfied and engaged with their work and therefore less likely to experience some of these negative effects emotional empathy can cause. Lack of empathy is an emotional consequence that results in a lack of motivation to provide compassionate care. It is clear that more research is needed on supporting survivors of SVA with regard to the direct impact on empathy of HCPs.

Fernandez and Zahavi (2021) suggest that a lack of a defined conceptual framework for understanding empathy is contributing to the impact of empathy on nurses' wellbeing. There is a difference in empathising with the other to provide compassion, as opposed to trying to experience the same emotional response/feelings/moods/sensations which can lead to an embodied response. HCPs can empathise with the survivors by drawing upon theoretical knowledge, rather than pulling from their own emotional empathy. Fernandez and Zahavi (2021) suggest that it is central to the role of HCPs that they do not imagine what it must be like to be the service user but to support them to find their own voice in order to express and articulate their viewpoint without influence from the HCP.

Considering this approach, it could be suggested that the traditional 'put yourself in their shoes' approach to empathy is morally questionable for HCPs because it is impossible to do and as such will always inflict a sense of failure. This sense of failure becomes a professional measure of competence and contributes to self-assigned failure on the part of the HCP. Clearly, there is a need to define and establish professional empathy so that the HCPs can be aware of the impact their emotional response may have on themselves and their service users. In Dosdales' study (2023), survivors of SVA indicated that if the disclosure has been made and the nurse does not respond in a way the survivor had hoped (empathetic and therefore belief), regret immediately sinks in and the emotional impact on them is evident. This often contributes to survivors disengaging with the service and other services, demonstrating the importance of that initial response to disclosures from the HCP.

Hockenbury and Hockenbury (2007) suggest that emotional reactions are a complex psychological state that have three distinct components: a subjective experience, a psychological response and a behavioural or expressive response. These components affect the HCP and impact the SVA disclosure experience. For example, in *a subjective experience* – the HCP interprets the survivor's experience based on their understanding and concept of what rape is and is shocked whilst trying to empathise, anxiety about supporting the survivor develops; *the psychological response* – the HCP could feel anger and/or sadness; and the *behavioural or expressive response* – the HCP compartmentalises their emotional feelings to carry out their tasks, they call the police to report the rape or experience a desire to hug the survivor as an expressive response. The emotional impact of receiving rape disclosures for HCPs is complex, and appropriate support and resources are a big implication for future practice. Whilst during the disclosure there is a process of compartmentalising in order to undertake certain aspects of what they deem is their professional responsibility, it is clear that the empathy the HCP may experience at the time does not leave at the end of the consultation. Instead, emotional feelings attributed to the consultation can be experienced even years later (Dosdale, 2023), demonstrating the need for psychological support for HCPs post-SVA disclosure.

## Additional Risk Factors

According to Kinman (2021), there are a number of key risk factors, alongside supporting survivors of SVA, that are likely to impact negatively on the mental well-being of staff working in the health sector. These include levels of perceived and actual workload; the level of autonomy staff hold to perform their role; the demands of the role in terms of levels of intensity. Other risks relate to working patterns including long hours and the frequency and length of breaks, staffing levels. Others relate to organisations culture and include factors such as the quality, the impact of leadership and cultural factors such as relationships with colleagues, feeling valued and respected, as well as being treated fairly at work and having opportunities to develop. Those who have existing mental health problems are at increased risk, as are those staff who have lower levels of resilience, support mechanisms and ability to engage in self-care. It is also noted that individuals of minority ethnic origin are at greater risk of poorer mental well-being. Kinman (2021) suggests there is evidence that staff from these backgrounds are at greater risk of bullying and abuse in the workplace and that statistics show they experience high numbers of fitness to practice investigations by regulatory bodies than their peers.

Whilst it is acknowledged that many working in health and social care are at risk of poor mental well-being, key studies have focused on those providing care to individuals who have experienced domestic violence and abuse. Nimmo and Huggard (2013), for example, indicate that physicians providing care such as sexual abuse therapy are at greater risk of developing both compassion fatigue and vicarious traumatisation. A qualitative literature review by Christensen, Metcalfe and O'Reilly (2021) focused on emergency department nurses' experiences of supporting female domestic violence presentations. In this review, it was clear that many of the staff experienced significant emotional impact as a result of ongoing exposure to the vulnerabilities and experiences of those they were caring for. This was compounded by the felt need of staff to hold it together for the sake of the service user alongside feelings of devastation and helplessness. These feelings were explained by staff who do not always feel educated or trained well enough to provide appropriate support, along with the wider organisational factors such as not having enough time or resources to provide adequate care and support. Some staff described suppressing or avoiding emotional interactions with service users, and this was both a response to dealing with the trauma they were confronted by, as well as what was referred to as emotional immunity (compassion fatigue) that developed due to repeated exposure.

## Consequences in the Workforce

If it is not addressed, work-related stress and burnout can lead to serious consequences for the health of the individual. It is known to increase the risk of unhealthy behaviours such as poor diet, increased use of alcohol, as well as impacting general health and increasing risk of musculo-skeletal problems.

Overall, 30% of NHS absences are attributed to stress and burnout, and these result in a financial cost of £300–400 million per year (Kinman, 2021). There are also organisational consequences in terms of the increased likelihood of errors and poor performance at work (House of Commons Committees, 2021). In addition, burnout is noted to be a significant factor in relation to staffing levels, impacting not only staff absence but also staff retention and the likelihood of attracting new staff into the health and care sectors (The Kings Fund, 2022). Staffing shortages are widely considered to be at a crisis point across both the health and social care sectors. In the NHS, the latest data (September 2022) shows a vacancy rate of 9.7%, increasing from 7.9% the previous year; this equates to a total number of 133,446 vacancies (The Kings Fund, 2022). Of these vacancies, 9,053 were for medical posts and 47,496 were in nursing, again increasing from 7,855 to 39,991 since the previous year. Care England (2022), which is the largest and most diverse representative body for independent providers of adult social care in England has asked the government to intervene to address the workforce crisis in social care. In adult social care alone, there are over 55,000 vacancies. It is widely accepted that the challenges facing the care sector compound those in the health sector and as such, there is an urgent need to address both.

### Supporting Staff Well-Being

A supportive work environment is positive for everyone, and the relationships we have with our colleagues can impact physical and mental health and well-being, as well as team and organisational performance. This is particularly important in high-stress and high-pressure environments. The National Wellbeing Hub (2023) highlights the value of peer support in the workplace, whereby individuals can provide and receive informal support from each other.
   **Key suggestions are:**

- Make time for team activities, including formal and informal meetings and coffee breaks.
- Include colleagues who may be working from home/independently.
- Get to know each other, especially new colleagues. This will help you notice any changes in mood or behaviour.
- Sharing your own experiences can help others feel they are not alone.
- Listening can be powerful.
- Find out where to get support or to sign post if needed.

Many organisations, for example, NHS Scotland, are embedding resources such as the Psychological First Aid Kit (NHS Scotland, 2020) into their staff training. This provides important information to staff and reassures them that their well-being is important, as well as providing staff with information about how to support their colleagues. Key features include caring for immediate safety needs, protecting the individual from further threat and distress, providing comfort and consolation, providing information and support, considering services that can help and connecting the individual with social support. Measures such as this make a valuable contribution to workplace well-being.
   Whilst those working in caring professions are at higher risk of poor mental health and well-being, it must also be noted that many staff report being highly satisfied and engaged with their work (Kinman, 2021). Indeed, it is noted that for many, whilst supporting

service users in challenging circumstances can be stressful, it can also produce a sense of purpose, fulfilment, and as a result, have therapeutic benefits for the staff involved (Kinman, 2021); this is noted to be the case for many staff who support those who are/have experienced trauma and crimes such as domestic/SVA (Office for Victims of Crime, 2023).

International approaches to supporting those working in occupations where there is exposure to vicarious trauma refer to models of examining and conceptualising the impact, as well as considering the roles and responsibilities of organisations in supporting their employees. For example, the Office for Victims of Crime (2022) outlines a model whereby exposure is thought to produce a change in worldview for many. This is considered an inevitable response where the individual can become more cynical or fearful or more appreciative of what they have. Both have the potential to considerably impact mental and emotional well-being (Anderson et al., 2019). The evidence suggests that there is a significant benefit to healthcare employees having access to and engaging with peer support and access to psychotherapies (Anderson et al., 2019). However, access to this needs to be consistent and not ad hoc or emergency-driven.

Many healthcare organisations have employee assistance programmes or occupational health departments whereby staff can often access health or psychological well-being. However, this is often in their own time and may involve a level of disclosure to managers or other colleagues that staff may be uncomfortable with, often causing barriers to accessing support. If this is the case, it is worth contacting your occupational health department directly and asking about their confidentiality policy. Many organisations now use third-party providers to deliver psychological well-being support to staff.

Clinical supervision has been used in healthcare practice for numerous years and is often focused on providing a safe space for the reflection of difficult cases and situations that HCPs may have encountered. It is also widely used as evidence for revalidation purposes to demonstrate critical thinking and improve the quality of care. Clinical supervision for HCPs is a structured and supportive process aimed at enhancing the quality of patient care and promoting professional development among HCPs. It involves regular meetings between a supervisor and a supervisee, where the supervisee discusses their clinical practice, challenging cases, reflects on their experiences and receives guidance and feedback from the supervisor.

Whilst a range of evidence validate its benefits (Brunero and Stein-Parbury, 2008; Susman-Stillman, 2020), the difficulty with clinical supervision is often regularity of access, and barriers of (frequently) managers, providing the clinical supervision which may impact how open and honest an employee may be. It is therefore important to note that clinical supervision is different from line management or performance appraisal. While supervisors may have some managerial responsibilities, the focus of clinical supervision is primarily on professional development and improving patient care.

## Self-Care

It is important to recognise the things that practitioners can do to protect and improve their own well-being and resilience. Caring for ourselves is vital in order that we may care for others. Key strategies include taking care of our own physical and social health by eating and sleeping well, taking regular exercise and getting adequate rest and time away from work. What is equally important is being kind to us and practising what is referred to as self-compassion (Vachon, 2016). Self-compassion is how we relate to ourselves in times of perceived failure, inadequacy or personal suffering (Neff, 2011). Very often we are prone to self-criticism, self-judgement, feelings of isolation or alienation and becoming consumed with our mistakes. What Neff (2011) suggests is that instead we treat ourselves with self-kindness and recognise our common humanity. What also helps is mindfulness whereby being present in the moment can help to bring about perspective and increase our ability to see things as they are without judgement. Self-awareness is an important way of building resilience, and it is important that practitioners acknowledge feelings of fear, anxiety, guilt, sadness and grief and accept that these emotions are normal responses to demanding and traumatic situations (Hofmeyer, Taylor and Kennedy, 2020).

## Suggestions for Organisations

Organisations play a key role in providing a culture that promotes and supports staff well-being. It is not surprising that the NHS, as one of the largest employers in Europe, and also an organisation where staff are exposed to the trauma of others, has developed policies and approaches to support staff. Indeed NHS England (2020) outlined the need to look after our people and keep staff safe, healthy and well, both physically and psychologically. The role of organisations in supporting well-being is extensive and relates to many organisational policies and procedures. Key measures include the need to consider working patterns, staffing levels, work-life balance, education and training and resources (Royal College of Nursing, 2021). This has seen the introduction of systems whereby individuals and teams are more supported. One example is the emphasis on communication rounds where staff can have time to discuss experiences and approaches to service delivery as well as wobble rooms. These are places where staff can go for a few minutes to share worries, express their emotions or sit quietly. The idea behind wobble rooms is that they create a culture where staff feel they can express emotions without judgement and can receive compassionate support. Other measures include the introduction of well-being champions to ensure staff are aware of support and services (NHS Leicestershire Partnership, 2020).

It is important that those in senior roles, including line managers, have regular and open conversations about well-being with their staff. This provides an opportunity to develop relationships where staff feel they can raise any concerns, and by getting to know colleagues, it is easier to identify any signs that might indicate the individual is having a negative response to exposure to trauma or may need further support. Senior staff can ensure that employees are aware of the support available to them and make sure this is publicised via organisational intranet sites and other modes of communication, as well as ensuring interventions such as Psychological First Aid are embedded in organisational training. Many organisations now have frameworks and best practice pathways to ensure that there is a clearly articulated and managed approach to supporting staff. A good example of this is St Mungo's Pathway for Staff exposed to a traumatic incident at work (2021).

## Trauma-Informed Approaches to Support Staff

Trauma-informed approaches (TiA) are essential to supporting healthcare staff who may be exposed to traumatic situations or who may have experienced trauma themselves (definitions of TiC&P can be found in Chapter 9) (Bateman, Henderson and Kezelman, 2013; Beattie et al., 2019). These approaches aim to create a safe and supportive environment that acknowledges and responds to the impact of trauma on individuals. Some of the key elements of TiA for supporting HCPs are:

- Education and awareness: Healthcare organisations should provide training and education to staff about trauma, its effects and the principles of trauma-informed care (TiC). This helps raise awareness and understanding of trauma-related issues and promotes empathy and sensitivity towards both patients and staff.
- Safety and trustworthiness: TiA contributes to creating a physically and emotionally safe work environment where healthcare staff feel secure and supported. This involves clear policies and procedures, respectful communication and a culture that prioritises psychological safety. Thus, improving health outcomes and therefore retention of staff.
- Emotional support and self-care: Provide resources and support for healthcare staff to address their emotional well-being and self-care needs. This can include access to counselling services, debriefing sessions, peer-support programs and self-care workshops. Encourage staff to take breaks, engage in stress-reducing activities, and seek support when needed.

In order to implement TiA in healthcare organisations, there needs to be support at a senior strategic level, as providing a TiC organisation will also involve reviewing and adapting organisational policies and practices to align with trauma-informed principles. This may include revisiting protocols for handling traumatic situations, addressing secondary trauma and burnout, and implementing trauma-informed screening and assessment tools.

Providing and committing to trauma-informed supervision for healthcare staff demonstrate that organisations are committed and focused on the emotional well-being, professional development, and support needs of their healthcare staff. Supervisors should be trained in TiA and be able to provide guidance, feedback, and resources to support staff in their roles. By implementing TiA, healthcare organisations can create a supportive and compassionate work environment that recognises and responds to the unique needs of healthcare staff who may have experienced trauma or work with trauma-affected individuals. This, in turn, promotes staff well-being, reduces burnout, and enhances the quality of care provided to patients.

## Compiling Statements

One of the potential consequences of not only supporting survivors of SVA, but also working in healthcare, is the risk of your notes being called to provide evidence in an inquiry, coroners or criminal court. This could be in the form of medical/nursing records and/or a statement being requested to use as evidence in any legal proceeding. In the field of health and social care, there are a variety of reasons why you might be asked to write a witness statement and it is understandable that this can be a daunting and anxiety-producing experience. It is not, therefore, unusual for you to be worried about the prospect of writing a statement. A 'compelled statement' gives certain authorities, such as the police, the power to require any person whom they have reasonable cause to believe will be able to provide information relevant to an examination or investigation, to answer such questions as the authorities have thought fit to as, and to sign a declaration declaring your statement to be true.

If the incident you are asked to write about is to be investigated, then the statement would form part of the investigation contributing to the defence or accusation of those involved. It is therefore very important that the statement is truthful and that it has been given much thought. Both your organisation and your professional unions will provide support for writing statements. The Royal College of Nursing (RCN) provide excellent guidance on this that could be transferable to any healthcare professional (https://www.rcn.org.uk/Get-Help/RCN-advice/statements).

When preparing a statement, it is always a good idea to get support from your employer and a trade union, but you must be very careful not to let such support interfere in any way with the truth and accuracy of your statement, for which you alone are finally responsible.

The first part of this process is your original record-keeping. Clinical documentation is record keeping for your protection and that of the service user. Documentation aims to:

- Provide notes which will justify your reasoning and decision-making further down the line
- Promote your coherent decision-making and reasoning

There are many situations whereby statements may be requested of you, below are examples of those:

- You are under investigation due to a complaint made against your practice or character. You could be asked for a statement following an adverse incident at work that you were directly involved in. For example, you may have administered the wrong dosage of medication to a patient, or you've been accused of unprofessional behaviour.
- Inquest/coroners court. If you have been involved in providing direct care to a service user in the period before an unexpected death. If you are asked to provide a statement for an inquest or coroner's court, check your employer's policy. You may be required to talk to your manager and/or employer's solicitor, before speaking to the Coroner's Office/officer. The policy should outline whether your employer will arrange representation for you to avoid potentially incriminating yourself.
- If there is a risk of you being prosecuted in connection with a death, you may have contributed in some way to the death, or you are concerned your practice might be criticised.
- A service user you have provided direct care to has disclosed an incident to you that is against the law or becomes the source of an investigation, such as SVA.

A witness statement is a signed document that records the evidence of the signatory, it is signed as confirmation that the contents of the document are true (Health & Safety Executive, 2023). The purpose is to provide support to either party during an investigation and, in some cases, disciplinary hearings. It has to be remembered that a witness statement is a legal document, and as such it can be used as evidence during investigations, at disciplinary hearing and also at later hearings. It has to be reiterated that in a witness statement, you must always provide a truthful and accurate report of the event.

It can be very frightening to be questioned by the police. If you are a suspect (i.e., the police say that they will be interviewing you under caution), you should not answer questions or submit any statement until you have legal support. If you are asked to be questioned as a witness, you should also seek support from your organisation and/or your professional union body.

**If you are asked to give evidence in any investigation the following may help you plan:**

- Take your time, speak slowly and clearly.
- Ask for the question to be repeated if you do not understand it or cannot hear.
- If you are not sure of the answer, say so.
- You can ask the judge for guidance.

Things to remember if you are asked for a statement or to give evidence in court:

- Seek support.
- Be factual.
- Most healthcare professionals called to give evidence don't get as far as the courtroom, most lawyers accept the evidence and don't need to question it.
- Court appearances are rare, which is why they are so nerve-racking (unless you are an expert witness).

## References

Anderson, E. C., Carleton, R. N., Diefenback, M and Han, P. K. (2019) 'The relationship between uncertainty and affect', *Frontiers in Psychology*. https://doi.org/10.3389/fpsyg.2019.02504

Bateman, J., Henderson, C. and Kezelman, C. (2013) Trauma-informed care and practice: Towards a cultural shift in policy reform across mental health and human services in Australia. A national strategic direction. Position Paper and Recommendations. Lilyfield, Mental Health Coordinating Council. Volume28, Issue1–2 January 2019 Pages 116–124

Beattie, J., Griffiths, D., Innes, K. and Morphet, J. (2019) 'Workplace violence perpetrated by clients of health care: A need for safety and trauma-informed care', *Journal of Clinical Nursing*, 28(1–2), pp. 116–124.

Brunero, S. and Stein-Parbury, J. (2008) 'The effectiveness of clinical supervision in nursing: An evidenced based literature review', *Australian Journal of Advanced Nursing*, 25(3), pp. 86–94. https://www.ajan.com.au/archive/Vol25/AJAN_25-3_Brunero.pdf

Care England (2022) Government Intervention Needed to Curb the Workforce Crisis in Social Care. Available at: https://www.careengland.org.uk/government-intervention-needed-to-curb-the-workforce-crisis-in-social-care/

Cavanagh, N., Cockett, G. and Doig, C. J. (2019) 'Compassion fatigue in healthcare providers: A systematic review and meta-analysis', *Nursing Ethics*, 27(3), pp. 639–665. https://doi.org/10.1177/0969733019889400

Christensen, M., Metcalfe, L. and O'Reilly, R. (2021) 'Emergency departments nurses experiences of female domestic violence presentations: A review of the qualitative literature', *Nursing Forum*, 56(4), pp. 771–1051. https://doi.org/10.1111/nuf.12632

Dosdale, C. (2023) *Adult experiences of rape disclosures in nursing practice: A phenomenological study*. PhD Thesis. Northumbria University. Available at: https://nrl.northumbria.ac.uk/id/eprint/51579/

Duarte, J., Pinto-Gouveia, J. and Cruz, B. (2016) 'Relationships between nurses' empathy, self-compassion and dimensions of professional quality of life: A cross-sectional study', *International Journal of Nursing Studies*, 60, pp. 1–11. https://doi.org/10.1016/j.ijnurstu.2016.02.015. Epub 2016 Mar 4. PMID: 27297364.

Fernandez, A. and Zahavi, D. (2021) 'Empathy in nursing: A phenomenological intervention', *Tetsugaku*, 5, pp. 23–29.

Health & Safety Executive (2023) Witness Statements Available at: https://www.hse.gov.uk/enforce/enforcementguide/investigation/witness-witness.htm#P1_48

Health and Social Care Committee (2021) The Scale and Impact of Workforce Burnout in the NHS and Social Care. Available at: https://publications.parliament.uk/pa/cm5802/cmselect/cmhealth/22/2205.htm#_idTextAnchor004

Hochchild, A. R. (2003) *The Managed Heart: Commercialization of Human Feeling, Twentieth Anniversary Edition, With a New Afterword*. Berkeley: University of California Press.

Hockenbury, D. and Hockenbury, S. E. (2007) *Discovering Psychology*. New York: Worth Publishers.

Hofmeyer, A., Taylor, R. and Kennedy, K. (2020) 'Knowledge for nurses to better care for themselves so they can better care for others during the Covid-19 pandemic and beyond', *Nurse Education Today*, 94. https://doi.org/10.1016/j.nedt.2020.104503

House of Commons Committees (2021) How Can We Tackle Staff Burnout in the Health and Care Sectors? Available at: https://houseofcommons.shorthandstories.com/health-and-care-staff-burnout/index.html

Joinson, C. (1992) 'Coping with compassion fatigue', *Nursing*, 22(4), pp. 118–119.

Kinman, G. (2021) Managing Stress, Burnout and Fatigue in Health and Social Care. Available at: https://www.som.org.uk/Managing_stress_burnout_and_fatigue_in_health_and_social_care.pdf

Kinman, G. and Teoh, K. (2018) What Could Make a Difference to the Mental Health of UK Doctors? A Review of the Research Evidence. Available at: https://www.som.org.uk/sites/som.org.uk/files/What_could_make_a_difference_to_the_mental_health_of_UK_doctors_LTF_SOM.pdf

Kinman, G., Teoh, K. and Harris, A. (2020) The Mental Health and Wellbeing of Nurses and Midwives in the United Kingdom. Available at: https://www.som.org.uk/sites/som.org.uk/files/The_Mental_Health_and_Wellbeing_of_Nurses_and_Midwives_in_the_United_Kingdom.pdf

McKinley, N., McCain, R. S. and Convie, L. (2020) 'Resilience, burnout and coping mechanisms in UK doctors: A cross-sectional study', *BMJ Open*, 10, p. e031765.

Moudatsou, M., Stavropoulou, A., Philalithis, A. and Koukouli, S. (2020) 'The role of empathy in health and social care professionals', *Healthcare (Basel)*, 8(1). https://doi.org/10.3390/healthcare8010026

National Wellbeing Hub (2023) How Can I Support My Colleagues? Available at: https://wellbeinghub.scot/resource/how-can-i-support-my-colleagues

Neff, K. (2011) *Self-Compassion*. New York: Harper Collins Publishers.

NHS England (2020) We are the NHS: People Plan for 2020/2021 – Action for Us All. Available at: https://www.england.nhs.uk/wp-content/uploads/2020/07/We-Are-The-NHS-Action-For-All-Of-Us-FINAL-March-21.pdf

NHS Leicestershire Partnership (2020) Positive Impact of "Wobble Rooms" on Staff Wellbeing Recognised Ahead of Mental Health Awareness Week. Available at: https://www.leicspart.nhs.uk/news/wobble-rooms/

NHS Scotland (2020) Psychological First Aid. Available at: https://wellbeinghub.scot/wp-content/uploads/2020/05/COVID-19-Psychological-First-Aid-7-slides-2.pdf

NHS Staff Survey (2021) NHS Staff Survey 2021. Available at: https://www.nhsemployers.org/articles/nhs-staff-survey-2021-results

Nimmo, A. and Huggard, P. (2013) 'A systematic review of the measurement of compassion fatigue, vicarious trauma, and secondary traumatic stress in physicians', *Australasian Journal of Disaster and Trauma Studies*, (1), pp. 37–44. http://tur-www1.massey.ac.nz/~trauma/issues/2013-1/AJDTS_2013-1_Nimmo.pdf

Office for Victims of Crime (2022) What Is Vicarious Trauma? Available at: https://ovc.ojp.gov/es/node/23636#:~:text=What%20is%20Vicarious%20Trauma%3F%20Vicarious%20trauma%20is%20an,continuous%20exposure%20to%20victims%20of%20trauma%20and%20violence

Ross, L. D. and Nisbett, R. E. (1991) *The Person and the Situation: Perspectives of Social Psychology.* New York: McGraw-Hill.

Royal College of Nursing (2021) Healthy Workplace Toolkit. Available at: https://www.rcn.org.uk/Professional-Development/publications/healthy-workplace-toolkit-uk-pub-009-734

Santo, D. L., Pohl, S., Saiani, L and Battistelli, A. (2014) 'Empathy in the emotional interactions with patients. Is it positive for nurses too?', *Journal of Nursing Education and Practice*, 4(2), pp. 74–81.

St Mungo's (2021) St Mungo's Pathway for Staff Exposed to a Traumatic Incident at Work. Available at: https://cdn.mentalhealthatwork.org.uk/wp-content/uploads/2019/07/30101914/SM-Pathway-for-staff-exposed-to-a-traumatic-incident-at-work-FINAL.pdf

Susman-Stillman, A. (2020) 'Reflective supervision/consultation and early childhood professionals' well-being: A qualitative analysis of supervisors' perspectives', *Early Education and Development*, 31(7), pp. 1151–1168. https://doi.org/10.1080/10409289.2020.1793654

The Kings Fund (2020) Urgent Action Is Needed to Improve Working Conditions for Nurses and Midwives. Available at: https://www.kingsfund.org.uk/press/press-releases/urgent-action-needed-improve-working-conditions-nurses-and-midwives

The Kings Fund (2022) The Health and Care Workforce: Planning for a Sustainable Future. Available at: https://www.kingsfund.org.uk/publications/health-and-care-workforce

Trivedi, S. S. (2023) Big rise in nurses trying to take their own lives due to burnout. *Nursing Standard*. Available at: https://rcni.com/nursing-standard/newsroom/news/big-rise-nurses-trying-to-take-their-own-lives-due-to-burnout-195011

Vachon, M. L. S. (2016) 'Attachment, empathy and compassion in the care of the bereaved', *Grief Matters*, 19(1), pp.20–25. https://search.informit.org/doi/10.3316/informit.104678476754164

Wei, H., Aucoin, J., Kuntapay, G. R., Justice, A., Jones, A., Zhang, C., Santos, H. P., Jr and Hall, L. A. (2022) 'The prevalance of nurse burnout and its association with telomere length pre and during the Covid-19 pandemic', *PLoS One*, 17(23), p. e0263603. https://doi.org/10.1371/journal.pone.0263603

Williston, J. C. and Lafreniere, D. K. (2013) '"Holy cow, does that ever open up a can of worms": Health care Providers' experiences of inquiring about intimate partners Violence', *Health Care for Woman International*, 34, pp. 814–831.

# 10  Reflective Journal

### Introduction to Chapter

Reflection is a process of learning through everyday experiences and forms an integral part of undergraduate, post-graduate higher education and continuing professional development. For healthcare professionals who need to maintain a professional registration, it is essential to engage in reflection. Reflection focused on sexual violence and abuse (SVA) demonstrates you are a safe practitioner with safeguarding and patient safety at your core. It allows for you to explore communication, working in partnership with your service users, inter-professional working and adherence to guidance, policies and legal frameworks. Use these pages to document any cases you felt challenged you within this topic. Explore them (maintaining confidentiality) at your revalidation appraisals throughout your careers.

This reflective journal will be structured around Gibbs' Reflective Cycle (1988). A downloadable PDF version of this reflective journal can be found at www.routledge.com/9781032126241

### Reference

Gibbs, G. (1988) *Learning by Doing: A Guide to Teaching and Learning Methods*. Oxford, Further Education Unit Oxford Polytechnic.

DOI: 10.4324/9781003225461-10

Date.................................................................................................

Area of practice......................................................................................

1  Description (what happened)

.......................................................................................................

.......................................................................................................

.......................................................................................................

.......................................................................................................

.......................................................................................................

.......................................................................................................

2  Feelings (what were you thinking and feeling during and after this experience)

.......................................................................................................

.......................................................................................................

.......................................................................................................

.......................................................................................................

.......................................................................................................

.......................................................................................................

3  Evaluation (what was good and bad about the experience, make sure to not only focus on the negative)

.......................................................................................................

.......................................................................................................

.......................................................................................................

.......................................................................................................

.......................................................................................................

.......................................................................................................

4 Analysis (what sense can you make of the experience, use supporting literature for depth)

.................................................................................................................................

.................................................................................................................................

.................................................................................................................................

.................................................................................................................................

.................................................................................................................................

.................................................................................................................................

5 Conclusion (based on your analysis, what else could you have done?)

.................................................................................................................................

.................................................................................................................................

.................................................................................................................................

.................................................................................................................................

.................................................................................................................................

.................................................................................................................................

6 Action (if the situation arose again, would you do anything differently? This formalises the action out of your reflection)

.................................................................................................................................

.................................................................................................................................

.................................................................................................................................

.................................................................................................................................

.................................................................................................................................

.................................................................................................................................

List any literature that guided your thoughts during this reflection:

.............................................................................................................................................

.............................................................................................................................................

.............................................................................................................................................

.............................................................................................................................................

.............................................................................................................................................

.............................................................................................................................................

# Index

Note: Page references in **bold** denote tables.

active listening 106–107
acute trauma 95
aftercare 104
Alexander the Great 8
anxiety 3, 5, 41, 53–54, 85–86, 111, 113–114,
    118–119
APPG for UN Women 39
assault by penetration 34
Asylum and Immigration Act 55
avoidance behaviours 95

behavioural/expressive response 114
blame 23–24; self-blame 24; and SVA
    disclosures 23–24
burnout 111; impact on healthcare staff
    111–112; NHS Staff Survey Data **112**
Butler, Josephine 51

Care Act of 2014 70
Care England 116
Centre for Disease Control and Prevention 100
Centre of Expertise on Child Sexual Abuse 66
children: born as a result of CRSV 84–85; and
    disclosures 25
Children Act 70, 105
Children and Social Work Act 70
child sexual abuse (CSA) 62–74; current
    situation 64–65; definitions and
    terminology 62–63; within digital
    context 65–67; family of victims
    and survivors 69; historical context
    in UK 63–64; impact of 68–70;
    indicators people present with and
    clinical considerations 67–68; legal
    position and policies response 70–71;
    organisations for help/support 71;
    overview 62; survivor 68–69, 71;
    victims 71; wider society 70
chronic trauma 95
clinical documentation 120
clinical supervision 117
communication 15, 22, 67, 105, 124

compassion fatigue 112–113
compelled statement 119–121
complex trauma 95
conflict-related sexual violence (CRSV)
    79–92; additional/national support
    organisations 90; causes and drivers of
    81; children born as a result of
    84–85; current situation 80–81;
    definitions and terminology 79–80;
    female genital mutilation 85–87;
    historical context 80; impact of
    83–84; individual/societal level factors
    82–83; in marginalised communities
    87–88; overview 79; prevalence 88–89;
    prevention of 87; ritual-related sexual
    violence/abuse 89–90; as strategy/
    military objective 83
consent: capacity 15; clear communication
    15; context of SVA 15–16; continuous
    15; equality 15; freely given 15;
    informed 15; non-verbal cues 16;
    respect for boundaries 15; revocable
    16; voluntary 15
consequences in workforce 115–116
Consultation on Child Abuse Prevention
    (1999) 63
Contagious Diseases Acts 51
COVID-19 pandemic 2, 39, 41
Crime Survey for England and Wales (CSEW)
    7; Office of National Statistics (ONS)
    65
Crown Prosecution Service (CPS) 55
cybersex trafficking 52
cyberstalking 40–41

Data Protection Act 70
depression 19, 111
digital empathy gap 67
digital trophies 67
disclosures: barriers to 19–20; blame 23–24;
    and children 25; defined 19; and
    diversity 24–25; hidden rape 22; and

men 25–26; positive and negative outcomes of 27; rape myths 20–22, **21**; screening for SVA 22–23; sexual violence and abuse 13–14, 19–27; unacknowledged rape 22
diversity and disclosures 24–25
durable goods 49

emergency medical needs 103
emotional numbness 96
emotional well-being 68
emotion dysregulation 96
empathy 113–115
End Violence Against Women (EVAW) Coalition 12–13
Equality Act 37, 88
European Convention on Human Rights (ECHR) 70
Everard, Sarah 38
'Everyone's Invited' 2
exploitation *see* sexual exploitation
externalising behaviours 68

family of victims and survivors 69
female genital mutilation (FGM) 85–87, 95
flashbacks/intrusive memories 95
forensic intervention 103
freedom of information (FOI) 11
freely given consent 15

GDPR 70

Health and Social Care Committee 111
healthcare practitioners (HCPs) 3–4, 50, 56; care for survivors of SVA 23; and rape myths 21; and self-blame 24; survivors' experiences of disclosing 26–27
health care professional (HCP) 98, 110, 113–115
healthcare professional reflective journal of practice 124
hidden rape 22
Human Rights Act 70
human trafficking: background and historical 51–52; current situation 52–53; defined 49; impact of 54–55; indicators people present with and clinical considerations 53–54; legal position and policies response 55–56; overview 49–50; supporting the individual 56; terminology and definitions 50–51; *see also* trafficking of people
Human Trafficking and Exploitation (Scotland) Act (2015) 55
hyper-arousal 96
hypervigilance 96

*Iliad* (Homer) 8
Indecency with Children Act 63–64

Independence Sexual Violence Advisors (ISVA) 102
Independent Commission for Aid Impact (ICAI) 80, 81, 83
Industrial Revolution 9
Information Sharing: Advice for Practitioners 70
informed consent 15
inquest/coroners court 120
internalising behaviours 68
International Abolitionist Federation 51
International Agreement for the Suppression of the White Slave Traffic 51
International Convention for the Suppression of the White Slave Traffic 51
International Criminal Court 79
Internet Watch Foundation (IWF) 67
interpersonal problems 96
interpersonal relationships 68
invisibility 88

lad culture 22
language and accessibility, survivors 89
legal parameters 105, **106**

marginalised communities: examples of 88; and poverty/homelessness 88–89; sexual violence and abuse in 79–92
medical and forensic care 103
men, and disclosures 25–26
mental health 26–27, 68, 99
Mental Health Act 105
'modern day slavery' 51
Modern Slavery Act (2015) 50, 55
Modern Slavery Human Trafficking Unit (MSHTU) 55
Murad Code 87

National Crime Agency (NCA) 2, 52, 55
National Institute for Health and Care Excellence 67, 71
National Referral Mechanism (NRM) 55
National Society for the Prevention of Cruelty to Children (NSPCC) 25, 64, 65
National Statement of Expectations (NSE) 12
National Wellbeing Hub 116
negative self-concept 96
negative self-perception 96
NHS England 118
NHS Long Term Plan 99
NHS Staff Survey Data 112, **112**
non-consensual sexual act 7
non-verbal cues 16

Offences Against the Person Act 9
Office for Health Improvement and Disparities 12
Office for Victims of Crime 117
Office of National Statistics (ONS) 10, 65

Office of the Children's Commissioner 70
Office to Monitor and Combat Trafficking in
    Persons 55, 56
Old Testament of the Holy Bible 8, 80
online sexual harassment 39–40, 67

Palermo protocol (Protocol to Prevent, Suppress
    and Punish Trafficking in Persons,
    Especially Women and Children) 51
perpetrators: police officers 13; sexual violence
    and abuse 13
physical health 41, 53, 68, 85
poacher 37
pornography 34, 49–50
post-traumatic stress (PTS) 19, 95–97, 113
poverty/homelessness 88–89
powerlessness 19–20
practitioner self-care guidance 110–121;
    additional risk factors 115; burnout
    111–112; compassion fatigue 112–113;
    consequences in workforce 115–116;
    empathy 113–115; organisations 118;
    overview 110; secondary traumatic
    stress 113; self-care 117–118;
    supporting staff well-being 116–117;
    trauma-informed approaches (TiA)
    118–119; vicarious trauma 113
prevalence: conflict-related sexual violence
    (CRSV) 88–89; of SVA 1–3, 9, 11–12,
    22–23, 37, 80
prevention of CSRV 87
Project deSHAME 67
prosecution rates 15
prostitution 49–52, 55, 79
The Protection of Freedoms Act (2012) 42
The Protection of Harassment Act of 1997 37,
    42
prowler 37
Psychological First Aid Kit 116
psychological response 114
public health 1, 3, 12

rape: defined 33; hidden 22; myths 20–22, **21**,
    27; unacknowledged 22
Rape Crisis England and Wales 10–11, 21–22
rape culture 22
*Rape Culture* 22
rape-related PTS (RR-PTS) 96
religious/spiritual beliefs 68
respect for boundaries, and consent 15
revocable consent 16
ritual-related sexual violence and abuse 89–90
Royal College of Nursing (RCN) 120

safeguarding 104–105
*Safeguarding Across the Life Span* (Keeling
    and Goosy) 104

Safeguarding Vulnerable Groups Act 70
satanic ritual abuse (SRA) 90
secondary traumatic stress 113
secondary victimisation/re-exposure to trauma
    98–99
self-blame 20, 24
self-care 117–118
self-compassion 117–118
Serious Organised Crime Agency 56
sexism and women 22
sex trafficking 50; impact of 54–55; individual
    54; wider society 54–55
sexual assault 7, 32–45; defined 32; historical
    context in the UK 36–37; legal
    definition of 33–34; types 32
Sexual Assault Referral Centre (SARC) 3
sexual assault referral centres 102
Sexual Discrimination Act (SDA) 37
sexual exploitation 50–51; trafficking of
    people for purpose of 49–58; WHO
    definition of 49
sexual harassment 32–33, 35; behaviours/
    actions included in 34; current context
    38–41; defined 34; historical context in
    UK 37; impact on family of survivors
    42; impact on society 42; impact on
    survivor 41–42; legal position and
    policies response 42–43; online 39–40
sexually transmitted infections (STI) 104
Sexual Offences Act 55
sexual violence and abuse (SVA) 1–4, 70;
    -associated PTS 3, 14; disclosures 13–14,
    19–27; historical context 8–10; impact of
    14; legal parameters 105; in marginalised
    communities 79–92; medical
    considerations **104**; overview 7; people
    who have experienced 8; perpetrators
    13; prevalence of 1–3, 9, 11–12, 22–23,
    37, 80; recent data 10–13; ritual-related
    89–90; social cost 14–15; supporting
    survivors of 95–108
sex workers 51
shame 20, 24, 25, 53
Simon, Andrea 13
social cost: prosecution rates 15; sexual
    violence and abuse 14–15
social withdrawal and isolation 96
socio-economic 68; boundaries 70; conditions
    82; groups 63; pressures 82
staff well-being 116–117
stalking 33; defined 35; historical context
    in the UK 37–38; impact on family
    of survivors 42; impact on society
    42; impact on survivor 41–42; legal
    position and policies response 42–43;
    surveillance 40; types of perpetrators
    36; types of survivors 35

stereotypes 88; gender 26; marginalised survivors 89; rape myth 11

strategy/military objective, CRSV as 83

subjective experience 114

survivors: child sexual abuse 68–69, 71; defined 22; from ethnically diverse backgrounds 24; experiences of disclosing to healthcare practitioners 26–27; family of 69; healthcare practitioners' care of 23; organisations 107–108; practitioner self-care guidance in 110–121; sexual harassment impact on 41–42; stalking impact on 41–42; supporting 43–45, 71, 95–108

technology-facilitated sexual violence (TFSV) 39, 65

Trades Union Congress 38

trafficking of people: and organised crime 55; for purpose of sexual exploitation 49–58; *see also* human trafficking

Trafficking Victims Protection Act (TVPA), USA 51

'transportation' of people 50

trauma 95–96; acute 95; chronic 95; complex 95; responses 96–97; response to 97–98; secondary victimisation/re-exposure to 98–99

trauma-informed approaches (TiA) 99, 118–119; implementation 101–102; principles of **100–101**

trauma-informed care (TiC) 99, 119; goal of 101

trauma-informed care and practice (TiCP) 99–102; *see also* active listening

trauma-informed practice (TiP) 99

UK Human Trafficking Centre (UKHTC) 55–56

unacknowledged rape 22

UN High Commissioner for Human Rights 81

UNICEF 62

United Kingdom (UK): child sexual abuse 63–64; Department for International Development 87; historical context in 63–64; second wave of feminism in 10

United Nations (UN) 50; Convention on the Rights of the Child 70; Palermo protocol (Protocol to Prevent, Suppress and Punish Trafficking in Persons, Especially Women and Children) 51; Security Council resolution 1325 79

United Nations Entity for Gender Equality and the Empowerment of Women (UN Women) 84

United States (US): second wave of feminism in 10; Trafficking Victims Protection Act (TVPA) 51

unwanted sexual behaviour 67

vicarious trauma 113

victim blaming: assumptions 20–22; defined 20

victims: child sexual abuse 71; family of 69; supporting 71

violence against women and girls (VAWG) 7, 10–13, 80, 82–83, 87

violence against women (VAW) movement 51

voluntary consent 15

vulnerability to re-victimisation 69

What Works to Prevent Violence against Women and Girls Programme 87

women's rights movement 50

Working Together to Safeguard Children 71, 87

work-related stress 111, 115

World Health Organisation (WHO) 49, 62–64, 86

World War 1 10, 63